Introduction

The Muscular Skeletal System Treated Naturally is part of a series which goes through the different body systems, covering all the main common problems that we as humans may have to deal with in our lives. As time prods us along and we start getting old and don't feel so immortal anymore, we will all get into trouble at some time and for the unlucky ones it could be serious. A lot of us have been failed by modern medicine especially through the system and the costs, along with hospitals always being fill, with long waiting times. This series is designed to empower you, educate you, help you prevent conditions getting worse, and give you the knowledge you need to know and hopefully make you able to have a good understanding of your condition, when you need to see your doctor. In this book I give to you all the Herbal and Homoeopathic remedies to the conditions you see in the first part of the index, and we have a good look at the really hard ones such as **Fibromyalgia and Carpal Tunnel Syndrome** along with the usual conditions of aging such as Arthritis and Rheumatism. We also show you some of the tricks athletes use to fast heal sprains and strains along with all that is mentioned in the index. For good health you have to take the best from both worlds especially nutrition. Next we move on to the diet you need to look at for this system especially for certain diseases, adding also the Superfoods for that system, and nutritional supplements that may also help you. Next you will come to the main herbal which will give you a very in depth write up about the herbs along with Precautions, Contraindications and the usual dosages. Following that is The Introduction to Herbal Medicine followed by Understanding Homoeopathy. There is more to medicine then just taking drugs, with common sense being the best medicine there is. When your body tells you there is something wrong pay attention and don't let it get worse. Then there are others like me who suffered from an Industrial Accident and still suffer decades later, and only God knows how many suffered road accidents. But that's life and the reality is you have to pick up the pieces and carry on. I hope these books make your life easier.

Mark Gilberd

Medical Herbalist, Homoeopath and Iridologist

Cover Picture supplied by yoksel zok of **Unsplash**

Pansy is one of our main remedies used in Rheumatism

The Musculoskeletal System

Diet and Nutrition for the Muscular Skeletal System

Herbs for the Muscular Skeletal System

(In alphabetical order)

The Musculoskeletal System
Aging and the Musculoskeletal System

From about the age of 30 the density of bones slowly begins to diminish. This loss of bone density accelerates more in women after menopause resulting in bones becoming more fragile which are more likely to break especially in old age. As people age the cartilage inside a joint becomes thinner which may make the joint less like a shock absorber as it used to be and less resilient and more susceptible to damage. In some people the surfaces of the joints do not age well especially in those who have done hard physical labor most of their life's which leads them to the early onset of Osteoarthritis. Joints can also become stiffer because the connective tissue within ligaments and tendons becomes more rigid and brittle. This change also limits the range of motion of the joints. Loss of muscle starts around the 30s and progresses throughout life with the amount of muscle tissue and the number and size of muscle fibers gradually decreasing. The mild loss of muscle strength places increased stress on certain joints such as the knees and the wrists but this can be partially overcome or at least significantly delayed by regular exercise. Muscles provide the force and strength to move the body under the coordination of the brain but this can be affected by changes in or damage to the nervous system and the muscles and joints themselves. Changes in the muscles, joints, and bones will affect the posture and walk as we continue to age and lead to weakness and slowed movement. The skeleton provides support and structure to the body. Joints are the areas where bones come together and are the weak spot of the system as we age because damage in one area creates problems and maybe damage in another area. A good example is the spine which is made up of bones called vertebrae. Between each bone is a gel like cushion called a disk which with age becomes smaller and shorter as the disks gradually lose fluid and with wear become thinner. The vertebrae also loose some of their mineral content making each bone thinner. The spinal column in some, especially old women become curved and compressed. Bone spurs caused by aging along with use and wear of the spine may also form on the vertebrae causing pain and dysfunction especially if they are crushing a nerve. The long bones of the arms and legs become more brittle because of mineral loss but they do not change length which makes the arms and legs look longer when compared with the shortened trunk. The foot arches become less pronounced contributing to a slight loss of height. The joints become stiffer and less flexible. Fluid in the joints may decrease along with the cartilage as joint capsules become worn and damaged. Minerals may deposit in and around some joints especially the shoulder. Hip and knee joints may begin to lose cartilage and degenerative changes begin to happen and get worse. The finger joints lose cartilage and the bones thicken slightly. Finger joint changes are most often bony swelling called entophytes and are more common in women. These changes may be inherited. Lean body mass decreases. This decrease is partly caused by muscle tissue atrophy. The speed and amount of muscle changes seem to be caused by genes and through life style along with hard physical labor which can wear the body out much sooner. Muscle changes often begin in the 20s in men and in the 40s in women. The muscle fibers shrink and tissue is replaced and repaired more slowly. Lost muscle tissue may be replaced with a tough fibrous tissue. This is most noticeable in the hands which may look thin and bony. Muscles are less toned and less able to contract because of changes in the muscle tissue and normal aging changes in the nervous system. Muscles may become rigid with age and may lose tone even with regular exercise.

Common Changes that Happen in Aging

Osteoporosis is a common problem especially for older women.

Bones become more brittle and may break more easily.

Compression fractures of the vertebrae can cause pain and reduce mobility.

The posture may become more bent and stooped.

Overall height decreases because the trunk and spine shorten.

Risk of injuries increases because of instability and loss of balance.

Breakdown of the joints can lead to pain, stiffness and deformity.

Joint changes affect almost all older people.

Movement slows and may become limited.

The walking gait becomes slower and shorter.

Walking may become unsteady and there is less arm swinging.

Older people get tired more easily and have less energy.

Some older people have reduced reflexes.

Strength and endurance change.

Loss of muscle mass reduces strength.

For Prevention and Delay

Being overweight is one of the worst problems that a worn out joint has to bear so now maybe is the time to get rid of the weight and make other necessary changes so as to make your future less painful and more enjoyable. Exercise is one of the best ways to slow or prevent problems with the muscles, joints, and bones. Design a moderate exercise program suited to you so as to help you maintain strength, balance, and flexibility. Exercise also helps the bones stay strong. Change your diet and get it focused on you and your conditions for example women need more calcium and vitamin D then men and also at this age diabetes can become a problem and start causing nerve and circulation damage.

Osteoarthritis

A progressive degenerative disease due to aging and wear and tear which largely affects the cartilage of load bearing joints causing thinning and wearing out and the development of bony spurs. The disease has a slow onset for some and can come on fast for those who overwork the body with a lot depending on the trade you have worked in throughout your life. Usually the large load bearing joints will wear out first followed by the smaller ones with exception usually being from genetic inheritance. The condition usually starts with tenderness and swelling of joints and bony swellings due to overgrowth of bone, pain and stiffness with movement and limitation of joint movement with maybe the presence of grating sensation or cracking when the joint is moved. Cartilage does not have a blood supply and gets nutrition through the synovial fluid so if there is injury to the joint capsule it may turn into a degenerative wound so always seek help. Immobilization does not really help as it is a case of use it or loose it. When repair processes fail to keep pace with degenerative changes osteoarthritis ensures. In men it most commonly affects the knees, feet and the spine while in women it is the fingers, hands, knees and spine. In the under 45 age group prevalence is greater in men but over 45 it is women. Onset is gradual and localized to one or a few joints; pain is the worse after exercise followed by stiffness. The process of destruction is as follows. The first part of the joint to become affected is the cartilage which becomes worn and rough and may wear away altogether, as this happens the bone tries to renew the cartilage but only grows little fringes of bone around its rim called osteophytes or more commonly known as spurs. As the joint becomes worse the osteophytes irritate the synovial membrane causing inflammation which in turn makes the joint stiff, hot, swollen and painful. Degeneration carries on from here till the joint is useless and the only option is an artificial joint.

Nodal Osteoarthritis - More common in women especially around menopause but men can also get them especially if the hands have had a hard time during life and the fingers have had many injuries especially crush injuries. They usually pick on the joints at the end of the fingers and give off a nervy type of pain and can make the end of the finger look crooked. They can be very painful but over time they harden and the pain goes away. They are called Heberden's Nodes.

DISH also known as diffuse idiopathic skeletal hyperostosis

(DISH) or Forestier's Disease - This is considered a form of degenerative arthritis or osteoarthritis. However DISH is characterized by a unique flowing of calcification along the sides of the vertebrae of the spine. In other words imagine a single vertebrae as a candle, now light it and let it burn for a while. As the candle burns wax dribbles down the sides. This is what the vertebrae look like on the x-ray and what distinguishes it from other conditions such as ankylosing spondylitis. This disease can fuse vertebrae together in pairs in different parts of the spine or maybe any way it likes. It is commonly associated with inflammation and calcification of tendons at their attachments points to bone so think of heel and elbow attachments. This can lead to the formation of bone spurs and the loss of elasticity around tendon attachment to the bones. All DISH seems to want to do is fuse everything together. **Causes of Osteoarthritis -** Age, occupation wear and tear, stress or injury, nutrient deficiency, some have a genetic basis such as in post-menopausal women (calcium deficiency speeds up the process), and the stress and strains of being overweight. **Nutrition -** Use a Calcium supplement but one that the body can assimilate easy with a good example being one made from animal bones as this has been assimilated before by a living creature so we know it is water soluble. Most supplements are made from calcium carbonate which is not all that water soluble so if you can only find these crush them up to powder which will give the body the best chance of absorbing some of it. Supplement Magnesium and Manganese in the early stages to help prevent and slow down the progression of the condition. Try to find a calcium supplement that has these all together. A low Phosphate diet with fresh whole foods, high in Calcium, Magnesium, Vitamin A and Niacinamide (B3) has a fairly marked impact on the pain especially in the back while Manganese stimulates the cartilage forming enzyme and possible regrowth of cartilage. Chondroitan Sulfate and Glucosamine can help by stimulating the production of more cartilage. **The three below can usually be bought together in a powder form. This is very important as it allows for easy and fast assimilation into the body which is very beneficial and in the long run cost effective because you know this form of supplement is**

being easily digested.

Glucosamine Sulphate - Has many biological functions among which are its role as a stimulant and precursor to the proteins that form cartilage. As we age our ability to produce GS decreases and causes the cartilage to lose its water holding capability causing the cartilage to become dry and ineffective as a shock absorber, leading to pain. GS normalizes cartilage metabolism and prevents cartilage degradation. Stimulates the biosynthesis of the key structural components of cartilage (mucopolysaccharides) that are essential for healthy joint function and repair. Mucopolysaccharides also allow the cartilage to hold water which in turn acts as a shock absorber. GS also acts as a mild anti-inflammatory. Often prescribed with **Chondroitin Sulphate`** for its synergistic effects.

1. Combines with Chondroitin for effective joint repair.
2. Helps relieve the pain and inflammation of arthritis and joint injuries.

Chondroitin Sulphate - Occurs naturally in the cartilage where it participates in the matrix structure. CS protects cartilage from degradation by inhibiting elastase which is the enzyme responsible for the degradation of cartilage and increases the synthesis of proteoglycans which is a key structural component of cartilage. Together with GS, CS has been found to increase hyaluronate concentration and viscosity of synovial fluid increasing lubrication within the joints. Like GS, CS exerts only a mild anti-inflammatory action and for this reason both are usually given together with anti-inflammatory nutrients such as MSM and bioflavonoids in order to obtain faster pain relief. Vitamins C, E, B3, B5, and B6 are also valuable adjuncts to supplementation with GS and CS.

Methyl Sulfonyl Methane (MSM) - Is a naturally occurring source of organic Sulphur. The concentration of Sulphur in arthritic cartilage has been shown to be about one third the level of normal cartilage. Other beneficial effects of MSM are due to its ability to reduce inflammation and to inhibit pain impulses along nerve fibers. Can be of benefit in conditions of bursitis, tendonitis, tennis elbow and RSI. As we age the levels of MSM in the body decrease. The last three above are very important not only in arthritis but in first aid to damaged sprained and twisted joints. **Treatment** - Because there is no cure treatment is concentrated on alleviating the symptoms of pain, stiffness, reducing the inflammation and trying to prevent deformity, physical therapy and as a last resort surgery. When the condition is still mild and in the early stages paracetamol is usually supplied by Doctors and Chemists because of less side effects. In the latter more painful stages non steroid anti-inflammatory drugs commonly known as NSAIDS are the common treatment and preferred because they control the pain and reduce the inflammation though caution is needed because of the side effects they can produce especially in the elderly and people with allergies. **Herbal Treatment** - Topical applications can be a very important part of treatment and very useful for pain relief and improving general comfort levels and local healing. Below are different methods and formulas. The first one is a Liniment using essential oils to make the formula, if you add four or more reduce the mls proportionally. Wintergreen Oil is a common oil found in over the counter formulas for Arthritis and Rheumatism but usually does not have the health warning below. You do not have to use the exact formula, Wintergreen with the ginger or pepper would work well enough as the heat created by the pepper or ginger would force the Wintergreen into the body. Always remember the essential oils cross over into the blood as that is part of how they work.

Liniment or Rub
1 litre rubbing alcohol
Eucalyptus oil 10 mls
Peppermint oil 10 mls
Rosemary oil 10 mls
Ginger oil 10 mls
Black Pepper 10 mls
Thyme 10 mls
Wintergreen oil 10 mls – This oil can slow blood clotting, also avoid when using blood thinning medication.
Mix together and rub into effected area several times daily.

Cayenne and Glycerine Liniment

Mix equal parts of tincture and glycerine.

Do not use on broken or sensitive skin. Hot and burning liniment that relieves pain in cold aching joints and muscles.

Ginger Fomentation for painful joints.

Fomentation is a topical herbal preparation that allows herbs to be absorbed through the skin.

Ginger root grated fresh 100 grams

Simmer in 1 litre of water for 10 minutes, strain; soak cloths in hot water and place over joints making sure you don't burn the patient.

For Sprains, Pains, Rheumatism and Arthritis.

Ginger root 2 parts

Slippery Elm powder 1 part

Cayenne 1 part

Lobelia 1 part

Pour boiling water 10 times or more the weight of the herbs onto the herbs and simmer gently for 10 minutes. Strain and place hot soaked cloths over the affected areas. Follow this treatment by application of a liniment.

Diet is Important - Besides what was said in Nutrition people with Arthritis or Rheumatism have an acid problem, mainly a uric acid problem. A lot of acids also form from the inflammatory response of the body making problems worse. If your diet is full of sugar, processed foods and alcohol then your diet is acid to. It is time to go to the diet section and have a look at the Acid and Alkaline Chart and Diet. Before you go I will introduce you to the main herbal acid remover which you will probably be taking for a while. Celery Seed (the great acid remover). To start alkalizing your body straight away just add a little bit of lemon juice or apple cider to your cold water in the fridge. Remember never change your diet in a hurry take your time, investigate new foods, avoid processed foods and try to make a diet you like and will keep to. **The herbs that follow are being put together as the main formula that we will use for Osteoarthritis.**

Celery Seed

Apium graveolens

Actions - Anti-inflammatory, antimicrobial, anti-rheumatic, bitter, carminative, hypotensive, antispasmodic, diuretic, sedative.

Celery seeds are rich in powerful diuretic oils that cleanse the body of excess fluids and stimulate the kidneys to flush out uric acid and excess crystals that can cause many problems such as gout, arthritis and kidney stones. Detoxes the musculoskeletal system and used in the elimination of uric acid and waste products and also as a urinary antiseptic. It can also be useful in nervous restlessness and spasmodic tension. You can also use Celery Seed to help lower your blood pressure as it acts both as a diuretic and a vasodilator working in a similar way to pharmaceutical drugs known as calcium-channel blockers, but its diuretic action does not alter the ratio of sodium to potassium in the blood. Celery Seeds can have a calming and sedative affect due to limonene which acts as a mild tranquiliser and may help in treating anxiety, nervousness, mental stress and insomnia. Use caution in acute kidney conditions. Is a traditional Chinese medicine for hypertension, gout and diabetes. Useful in nervous restlessness and spasmodic tension, both topically and internally. **Contraindications** – Use with caution in acute kidney conditions due to the irritating effect of the volatile oils. Avoid in pregnancy and people with low blood pressure. **Part used** - Fruit (seeds) and root. **Constituents** - Volatile oil, limonene, Vitamins C, beta-carotene, sodium, magnesium and calcium, iron, potassium, zinc. **Dosage -** Tincture 2 to 4 mls 3 times daily. Infusion – 1 to 2 teaspoonful's of crushed seeds to cup of boiling water. Cover cup and infuse for 10 minutes 3 times daily.

Herbal Medicine regards Arthritis and especially Rheumatism as a deep seated chronic disease made worse by the buildup of waste products over a long period of time, meaning you are getting old. In other words injury, toxic overload and an aging body that doesn't work as good as it used to, needs a hand to take the weight off the main rubbish removing parts of the body, which are the digestive system especially the bowel which if constipated would be putting a large burden on the body especially the liver, the urinary system and especially the kidneys that has to remove all the uric acid and other waste products for which we will be using **Celery Seed** for. As we all know old age takes its toll on these systems so now is the time for a spring clean. I try to make most herbal formulas no more than five herbs and make them all work with each other for a common cause, if you go over 5 you tend to get lost but you can usually find 5 herbs that can work fairly well together, and emphasize and make stronger the main actions you want to use in the treatment of a condition. For our main remedy in our arthritis formula we shall use Devils Claw below which enhances some of Celery Seeds actions.

Devils Claw

Harpagophytum procumbens

Actions - Anti-inflammatory, anti-rheumatic, analgesic, sedative, diuretic, antioxidant, bitter and hepatic.

Specific for rheumatic and other joint diseases, arthritis, pain and muscle pain, lumbago, tendonitis, gout and inflammation of connective tissues. Devil's Claw is also beneficial in decreasing the progression of osteoarthritis by preventing cartilage degradation. Has a significant anti-inflammatory activity. Can also be used for tendonitis and to treat degenerative diseases of the musculoskeletal system. Affects the liver, stomach, joints, kidneys and is also a blood cleanser, removes deposits in joints, aids in the elimination of uric acid from the body. It is also a digestive tonic as the flavonoids and phytosterols found in Devil's Claw are antioxidant and stimulate bile production and is also an antispasmodic which may help in tummy cramps. The German Commission has given its approval on the Osteoarthritis and Digestive side. **Parts Used** – Secondary Tuber like roots. **Contraindications -** Caution with peptic ulcers and congestive heart failure. Not recommended during pregnancy or for diabetics, high doses can cause tummy upset. **Toxicity -** Higher doses may cause transient mild GIT disturbances such as diarrhoea and wind. **Interactions -** Less effective if taken with antibiotics (needs intestinal bacteria for activation). **Dosage -** As on bottle for capsules. 1 to 4mls of tincture 3 times daily.

Note how some of the actions are similar to Celery Seed especially the

Uric Acid one, this is because I want them to work together as a team, also I am using this herb for its action on the liver which is our main blood cleaner along with the kidney. Devils Claw bitter action will help stimulate and improve the digestive system. Devils Claw main job is to work on pain and inflammation. The next herb we add is Meadowsweet.

Meadowsweet

Filipendula ulmaria

Actions - Antiseptic, analgesic, anti-inflammatory, astringent, diaphoretic, anti-coagulant, acid balancer, carminative, anti-emetic, digestive, hepatic, anti-rheumatic.
One of the best digestive herbs and is also known as the acid balancer. Containing salicylic acid Meadowsweet is an effective herb against inflammation along with having with other compounds in it making it much easier on the lining of the stomach. Has specific use for peptic ulcers both as preventative and for treatment, especially the chronic ones. Meadowsweet has been shown to inhibit the growth of the Helicobacter pylori bacteria. Used for heartburn, hyperacidity, gastritis and reduces fever. Regulates gastric acid levels and protects and soothes the gastro intestinal tract and mucous membranes. Its gentle astringency is useful in treating diarrhoea, especially in children. Of great use in musculoskeletal conditions such as arthritis, gout and all kinds of muscle and joint pains. It promotes uric acid excretion. **Parts used** – Aerial. **Constituents** - Volatile oil, salicin, salicylic acid (analgesic and anti-inflammatory), flavonoids, tannins, coumarins, mucilage. **Contraindications** – Avoid if you are allergic to salicylates or aspirin. **Dosage** - Tea 1 to 2 tea spoonsful in cup of tea infuse for 10 minutes. Tincture 1 to 4 mls 3 times per day.

This herb in keeping with our intention is an acid balancer, pain killer and focuses on the digestive system. Next herb will be Willow Bark which is a very old herb in the treatment of arthritis and doubles our pain killing action with more salicin making this formula a useful pain killer to take at night for a more comfortable sleep.

Willow Bark

Alba

Actions - Analgesic, anti-inflammatory, febrifuge, bitter, astringent, antiseptic, anti-rheumatic.

Some people call this caveman's aspirin but the active chemical constituent salicin was only identified in 1829 by the French pharmacist H Leroux. This herb is used for a variety of conditions with the main symptoms being fever and pain. Salicin is a powerful anti-inflammatory and analgesic while other components of Willow bark have antioxidant, fever reducing, antiseptic and immune boosting properties. Used for mild flus and colds with fever, mild headaches and other pains caused by inflammation and used as a specific for Osteoarthritis and Rheumatism and other systemic connective tissue conditions with inflammatory changes such as anyklosing spondylitis, gout, muscular rheumatism, joint pain, osteoporosis, tendinitis, sprains, sciatica and neuralgia. This is also a good herb for heart health as it acts the same as aspirin but is longer lasting and it doesn't upset the stomach because it is absorbed into the blood via the large bowel so it prevents ulceration of the stomach and can be effective in reducing the risk of heart attacks and strokes. Antioxidant compounds called polyphenolic glycosides and flavonoids in willow bark have been shown to protect against oxidative stress and various symptoms tied to aging, such as poor physical performance, cognitive decline. **Pharmacology** - Salicin is analgesic and anti-inflammatory. Is metabolized to saligenin in the bowels, then absorbed and metabolized to salicylic acid. **Toxicity** – Do not take if you are allergic to salicylates. High doses may cause gastric and renal irritation. **Interactions** - Avoid with alcohol, barbitutates or other sedatives, NSAIDs and anticoagulants. **Parts used** - Bark (dried from 2-3 year old branches). **Constituents** - Mainly Salicylates with some others being beta-carotene rutin, tannins, calcium, iron, magnesium, manganese, phosphorus, potassium, selenium, zinc, B-vitamins, and Vitamin C. **Dose** – Tincture 4 to 7 mls 3 times daily. Infusion - Powder can be made into a tea, by infusing in boiling water for 10 minutes. Dosage 1 to 2 tea spoons of herbal powder to a cup of boiling water up to 3 times per day. Do not exceed the dosage, better to see how much less you can get away with, too much can upset the tummy.

Our final herb for this formula is Ginger which we are using for two reasons with the first being to push the formula into the body by its spicy heat and the second for its anti-inflammatory actions. Ginger could be replaced by Licorice for the same reasons but this herb uses its detergent properties to spread the formula along the small intestines to enhance absorption.

Ginger

Actions - Carminative, diaphoretic, circulatory stimulant, sialagogue, vasodilator, ant emetic, anti-inflammatory, antispasmodic and mild anti biotic.

Ginger may be used as a stimulant of the peripheral circulation in cases of bad circulation, chilblains and cramp. In feverish conditions ginger acts as a diaphoretic promoting sweat and cooling the body. As a carminative it promotes gastric secretions and is used in dyspepsia, flatulence and colic. Reduces cramping, gas and nausea. Used for motion sickness. Ginger is good to mix with any other combination of herbs because it would help the body to assimilate those herbs and increase their actions.

Doses - Used in teas, tinctures, powders in capsules and my favorite, crystallized Ginger which you can get in mild, medium or hot.

Examples of other Arthritis Formulas

Licorice - Anti Inflammatory also used to push formulas into the body
Devils Claw - As above,
Birch - Used more for its diuretic actions a little like Celery Seed.
Celery Seed - as above.
Feverfew - Anti Inflammatory and Digestive Bitter.
Guaiacum - Old remedy for Arthritis and Rheumatism. Made from plant resin.

Ginger - As above.

Humbert Santillow - Formula for Arthritis, RA and gout.
Chaparral 4 parts
Yucca 2 parts
Dandelion 1 part
Sassafras 1 part
Prickly ash 1 part
Black cohosh 1 part
Ginger root 1 part
Burdock root 1 part
The herbs are all finely powdered and packed into capsules.
Dose - take 2 to 3 times a day.

Note - Buying herbs in powder form is fairly easy these days especially in Australia. I buy most of mine from Queensland mostly from organic Herb farms which you can find a few of them on eBay. If you want to go this way then you will be happy to know that you can also buy capsule loading equipment that makes the job easier.

Homoeopathic Remedies for Osteoarthritis

Colchicum 6C to 30C - The typical case calling for Colchicum is where the swelling is red or pale, with extreme tenderness to touch, a tendency to shift about from joint to joint, and pains which are worse on the slightest motion. If the general symptoms of great prostration of the muscular system and abdominal bloating can be present Colchicum is the remedy. Gastric symptoms and cardiac complications also characterize. It is more indicated when the smaller joints, fingers, toes, wrists and ankles are affected; the pains are very violent, patient cannot bear to have the parts touched or to have anyone come near him. The Colchicum patient is apt to be exceedingly irritable and the gout is not apt to decrease this irritability.

Ledum 6C to 30C - Ledum is a useful remedy in gout as well as in many articular troubles. We have the symptoms that the ball of the great toe is swollen, sore and painful on stepping, drawing pains worse from warmth, pressure and from motion. It has also gouty nodosities in the joints, it differs from Bryonia in having a scanty instead of a profuse effusion; it is, perhaps, better adapted to hot swelling of the hip joint than is Bryonia. All the pains of Ledum travel upwards. Ledum, it must be remembered is a cold remedy, and attending all the symptoms is a general chilliness and lack of animal heat.

Ammonium Phos 6C to 30C - This is a useful remedy in constitutional gout where there are nodosities in the joints. It is not so much a remedy for the acute symptoms, but for chronic cases where there are deposits of urate of soda concretions in the joints and the hands become twisted out of shape.

Take a look at the remedies under Rheumatism

Rheumatoid Arthritis

Rheumatoid arthritis can happen at any age but is most likely to show up between the ages of 30 and 50. If it starts between the ages of 60 and 65 it's called elderly-onset Rheumatoid Arthritis which is different to the early one.

Early-Onset - Happens in young and middle-age adults. Among younger people women are more likely to get it. If you get RA when you're younger the symptoms tend to show up over time. With younger people the disease mostly starts in small joints like your fingers and toes. Around 80% of people with early-onset have Rheumatoid Factor which is the main culprit they look for in blood tests.

Elderly-Onset - Symptoms come on quickly in elderly-onset and men and women get it at nearly the same rate. People who get the disease later in life only make up about one-third of all people with the disease. Elderly-onset usually strikes large joints like shoulders and knees. Rheumatoid factor which is what they look for in the blood test to diagnose is less common in elderly-onset. If your blood tests show you have Rheumatoid Factor your disease will probably be more aggressive and severe than someone who doesn't. You can have elderly onset and osteoarthritis at the same time so you're Doctor needs to check you out fairly well and give you the needed blood tests. Elderly-onset Rheumatoid Arthritis can have symptoms that overlap with other diseases listed below.

Polymyalgia rheumatica
Late-onset psoriatic arthritis
Viral arthritis
Osteoarthritis
Hypothyroidism
Parkinson's disease

Early signs of Rheumatism are pain and swelling in the joints of the fingers and wrist but sometimes of the feet, shoulder, elbows, knees and even the jaw. Often the same joints in both arms and legs are affected at the same time. The joints are stiff and painful first thing in the morning with the stiffness wearing off gradually after an hour and getting better during the day. You may be felling generally unwell and feverish. Nodules which are usually found in areas of pressure are another sure sign of rheumatism they are movable, firm, rubbery and sometimes tender. These are the main leading symptoms of Rheumatism that distinguish it from Osteoarthritis. **Herbal Treatment** - I have decided to try a different approach for Rheumatism as I am angry that as my working life nears an end they still have no idea of what it is. What little we have is not very helpful such as it's an unknown autoimmune disease, maybe even a virus that tends to follow genetics that can attack other parts of the body, other than just the muscular skeletal system. Obviously a big part of the treatment must be tackling the uric acid side and getting rid of that along with all the wastes being made from the damage the disease makes. See the diet part of Osteoarthritis as the Acid Alkaline diet is very important here as you can very quickly see if you are loading your body with acids. Everything in the Osteoarthritis section is relevant to Rheumatism even the formulas so treat it as one big section. Now we have the diet being assessed it's time to get to the elephant in the room. We have been told that Rheumatism is an autoimmune disease so that means there must be something wrong with the immune system (I wonder how the virus feels about that). So the big question is have you ever had anything wrong with your immune system, have you had allergies, are you allergic to any foods, do you have asthma, do you have eczema or other skin reactions, or reactions to medications or anything. In other words it's time to see an Allergy Specialist to see if they can get you to react to anything or rule this out as it's an answer you must have for effective treatment and to avoid the wrong treatment. Gather all the information you can especially if it runs in the family, how severe was their condition? How were they being treated? Remember you only have 5 to 10 minutes of time with the Doctor before your medicated, so you have to give them as much information as you can. Now we are going to make a formula for Rheumatism like what we did for Osteoarthritis. We are going to replace Celery Seed with Pansy which like Celery Seed is a diuretic but has other actions such as a blood cleanser, allergy and works on autoimmune diseases. This will be our first allergy autoimmune herb which we are going to keep building up on. Note that we are also concentrating on the anti-inflammatory's and pain actions.

Pansy

Viola Tricolor

Actions - Analgesic, diuretic, anti-inflammatory, anti-pyretic, anti-allergic, expectorant, alterative, laxative, diuretic, vulnerary, anti-rheumatic.   Mostly used in three areas, the skin, lungs and urinary system. Specific for eczema and skin eruptions with exudates especially with rheumatic symptoms. Can be used both internally and topically for any skin disorder with purulent discharge, psoriasis, acne and also for autoimmune diseases and edema. Topical use for cradle cap, diaper rash, weeping sores, itchy skin (Chickweed), varicose ulcers and ringworm. As a diuretic can be used for dysuria associated with cystitis and as well as frequent and painful urination. Will also be of benefit in capillary fragility, easy bruising and atherosclerosis. For the respiratory system it will act as an anti-inflammatory expectorant for phlegm in the lungs, bronchitis and whooping cough. **Part Used** – Aerial. **Constituents** - Rutin, salicylates, zinc, saponins, mucilage, gum, resin. **Toxicity** - High doses may cause nausea and vomiting and allergic skin reactions. **Root** is emetic in high doses and has been used to induce vomiting in cases of poisoning. **Dose** - Tincture 2 to 4mls three times a day. Infusion 1 to 2 teaspoonful's of herb to boiling cup of water infuse 10 minutes.

For our second herb we will use Meadowsweet again as it is a good back up for Pansy especially in the acid removal area and by this time you should of changed the diet so there should be less acid going into the system.

Meadowsweet
Filipendula ulmaria
Actions - Antiseptic, analgesic, anti-inflammatory, astringent, diaphoretic, anti-coagulant, acid balancer, carminative, anti-emetic, digestive, hepatic, anti-rheumatic.
One of the best digestive herbs and is also known as the acid balancer. Containing salicylic acid Meadowsweet is an effective herb against inflammation along with having other compounds in it making it much easier on the lining of the stomach. Has specific use for peptic ulcers both as preventative and for treatment, especially the chronic ones. Meadowsweet has been shown to inhibit the growth of the Helicobacter pylori bacteria. Used for heartburn, hyperacidity, gastritis and reduces fever. Regulates gastric acid levels and protects and soothes the gastro intestinal tract and mucous membranes. Its gentle astringency is useful in treating diarrhoea, especially in children. Of great use in musculoskeletal conditions such as arthritis, gout and all kinds of muscle and joint pains. It promotes uric acid excretion. **Parts used** – Aerial. **Constituents** - Volatile oil, salicin, salicylic acid (analgesic and anti-inflammatory), flavonoids, tannins, coumarins, mucilage. **Contraindications** – Avoid if you are allergic to salicylates or aspirin. **Dosage** - Tea 1 to 2 tea spoonsful in cup of tea infuse for 10 minutes. Tincture 1 to 4 mls 3 times per day.

Nettles
Urtica dioica
Actions - Astringent, diuretic, tonic, galactagogue, tonic, nutritive,

anti-allergenic, anti-inflammatory, anti-septic, anti-hemorrhagic, hemostatic, hypotensive, nutritive, anti-rheumatic.

Is specific for nervous eczema and will strengthen and support the whole body. Plays an important role in chronic and degenerative conditions of the musculoskeletal system such as Rheumatism and Osteoarthritis, Gout, along with joint and muscle pain. A new study found Nettle Leaf extract had a positive effect against the genes associated with rheumatoid arthritis. Increases urine output and the removal of uric acid. The diuretic action makes it useful in the treatment of fluid retention, arthritis with swollen joints, and congestive heart disease. Specific for nervous eczema and children with eczema. Preventative against many ailments, hay fever, allergies, eczema and hemorrhage. Used in the treatment of wasting diseases, poor appetite, lung disorders, blood impurities and allergies. **Prostrate Problems** - Recent studies have found that Nettle is effective in reducing prostate size. It not only reduces the prostate size, it also alleviates the symptoms such as the frequent urge to urinate, painful urination and incomplete emptying of the bladder. Nettle leaf works well for inflammation of the prostate and other inflammations whilst the Nettle root is much better for BPH. Benign prostatic hyperplasia which means prostate gland enlargement. Nettles is an effective diuretic that can also help to break down stones in the kidney preventing painful conditions from worsening or requiring those stones to be either passed or surgically removed. **Precautions -** Hypersensitivity or allergy to Nettles may occur so start with a low dose. **Dose** - 2 to 4mls of tincture 3 times a day. Infusion 1 to 3 teaspoons full 3 times daily. Used as a tea from the leaf and or root. Taken in powdered root form for prostrate purposes.

Our next main herb is Cats Claw which works on allergies and has an action on the immune system a bit like an Adaptogen but what they are now calling an Immune modulator which means if it's an autoimmune response it will tone it down and if the body is slow on a disease threat it will speed it up. This herb is also anti-viral so it is the first attack on our hiding Rheumatism virus. More than any other herb this one really attacks on all fronts and multiplies the actions of our other herbs.

Cats Claw

Uncaria tomentosa

Actions - Anti oxidant, immune stimulant, anti-inflammatory, anti-fungal, anti-rheumatic, anti-viral, anti-tumor, anti-microbial.

Used to improve osteoarthritis and rheumatoid arthritis symptoms. Can help in reducing pain associated with activity. We are mainly using this herb because Rheumatism is an autoimmune disease, so you need to pay attention to what happens here, as it is working alongside Nettles which is the other herb we are using for the same reason. Traditional uses in Peru are as an anti-inflammatory, contraceptive and anti-cancer remedy. Can alleviate allergic sinus type conditions; boost the immune system, used for asthma, bursitis, Candida, immune deficiency disorders, chronic inflammatory diseases and auto immune conditions. This is a good herb for the Auto Immune types of diseases especially those that have an effect on the digestive system. An immune stimulant especially used in viral infections, including HIV. Useful in a variety of inflammatory diseases including gastric ulcers, diarrhea and GI tumors, gonorrhea, acne, diabetes, diseases of the urinary tract and cancer. A recent study showed that Cat's Claw significantly elevated the infection fighting white blood cell count in adult men who supplemented with this herb for 6 months. Researchers also noted a repair in DNA of both single and double strand breaks. Its effect on the immune system appears to be two fold, with the ability to both boost and dampen immune response (that's why we are using if for Rheumatism), depending on what is needed. Hyper immune responses can be contained, whilst a weak immune system that allows disease to advance undeterred is strengthened by supplementation with Cat's Claw. **Contraindications** -Pregnancy, lactation or in children less than three years old. **Interactions** - Typically not recommended for those taking insulin, thymus extracts, vaccines or immune globulin. **Precautions** - Do not take Cat's Claw if on blood thinning medication. Large quantities can cause stomach upset because of the large number of tannins in the bark. **Dose** - As labeled by supplier. Traditionally the bark of Cats Claw is made into a tea or powder to be consumed over a given period depending on illness.

For our 5th and last herb we are using Licorice. Licorice does the same job as Ginger in the last formula but in a different way. Ginger uses heat to push the formula into the body while Licorice has a detergent property which when it enters the fluid laden small intestines will spread the formula out allowing for faster and easier assimilation. Notice this herb is antiviral doubling our action here. The herb is a strong anti-inflammatory working in a similar way to the corticosteroids the Doctors give you but in a far gentler way. With this herb it will be only 10% of the formula as I mainly want it to force the formula into the body but I also want sympathetic actions to the cause to go along with it. Cats Claw and Nettles are our main herbs of the formula so choose the one that suits you better and we make this 30% of the formula. The remaining herbs will be at 20% each completing the formula. Herbalists usually work in Tinctures which are of a higher strength but you can also use the same percentages on powdered herbs and use for teas or put them in capsules.

Licorice

Glycyrrhiza glabra

Actions - Anti bacterial, anti-viral, expectorant, demulcent, anti-inflammatory, adrenal tonic, anti-spasmodic, mild laxative, nutritive. Licorice improves macrophage activity and increases the production of interferon which is antiviral. Licorice extract also has broad spectrum anti-microbial effects along with being an antioxidant protecting the tissues especially those of the liver from free radical damage. The root part is used, licorice is one of our best demulcents especially for sore throats and painful and inflamed airways where it hurts to cough and is also good for gastric ulcers as it coats and soothes them giving protection and reducing the inflammation, it is also nutritive and slightly laxative. It contains the building blocks of hormones, has a marked effect on the endocrine system and the glands of the body along with catarrh, bronchitis, coughs, gastric and peptic ulcers and abdominal colic. Can be used for treating inflammatory and allergic conditions. A recent study at the Institute of Medical Microbiology and Virology, Kiel, Germany, researchers found that licorice extract produced a potent effect against strains of H. pylori which are the main culprits for Peptic Ulcers. **Uses** - Treatment of cough, inflamed throat, pneumonia, pleurisy, TB, all catarrhal conditions, gallstones, chronic constipation, arthritis, fatigue, female infertility, pains of colic, stress, easing gastric ulcers, inhibits the herpes simplex virus. **Interactions** - With diuretics, cardiac glycosides, corticosteroids, blood pressure medications, laxatives. **Caution** - Do not use with high blood pressure. Long term use can also raise the blood pressure. Better for use in formulas, minimal adverse effects if intake is less than 10mg/day. **Dose -** 1 to 3mls of the tincture 3 times a day.

And now we come to my secret weapon which we will use as a supplement which is Borage. Use the oil which is usually sold as Starflower oil as a replacement for Fish Oils. This supplement has a strong action on toning down the immune and inflammatory response and is probably working as an adaptogen by adapting the body to what is happening and modifying the immune's systems response along with cleaning out the wastes which aggravate the situation.

Borage

Used as Starflower Oil

The oil which is what we will be using can be used to treat atopic dermatitis, dysmenorrhea, PMS, cyclic mastalgia, rheumatoid arthritis, hypercoagulative states, dyslipidemia, hyperlipidemia, hypertension and diabetic neuropathy. Borage Oil (more commonly known as Starflower Oil) is pressed from the seeds. **Starflower Oil Benefits** - Rich in Essential Fatty Acids - The seeds of this herb are comprised of roughly 25 percent oil which is one of nature's richest sources of gamma linolenic acid (GLA). GLA is a type of Omega 6 fatty acid which cannot be made by the body, requiring it to be obtained from outside sources. It is powerfully anti-inflammatory

and converts into beneficial prostaglandins, which have a profound reduction on the impact of inflammation on cardiovascular disease, lung function, autoimmune conditions and metabolic abnormalities.
Dose - Starflower Oil is typically taken in capsule form 1 to 4 daily.

Other Formulas for Rheumatism

Hoffman
Infuse 30g of the following dried herbs in 600mls of boiling water. Take 50 to 60 mls 3 times daily before meals.
Bogbean 2 parts
Black cohosh 1 part
Celery seed 1 part
Meadowsweet 1 part
Yarrow 1 part

Barkers Formula
FE Sarsparillia 30mls   FE means Fluid Extract
FE Guaicum 4mls
FE Bogbean 16mls
FE Yarrow 30mls
FE Lily of Valley 2ml
Concentrated Peppermint water 2mls
Add water to make 250 mls. Dose 20 to 50 mls every 4 hours.

Dominion College
Barberry bark 15g
Bogbean 15g
Yarrow 15g
Burdock 15g
Meadowsweet 15g
Raspberry 15
Simmer in 1.8 litres of water for 20 minutes. Add 30g of Licorice powder and infuse for 5 minutes. Strain while hot and add one teaspoon of Cayenne. Take 50 to 60 mls three times daily.

Homoeopathic Treatment for Rheumatism

Rhus Toxicodendron 6C to 30C - All Rhus rheumatic symptoms are relieved by motion. They are worse from sitting and worse from rising from a sitting position, or on first commencing to move; continued motion however, relieves. Warmth also relieves the Rhus rheumatism. Damp weather and the approach of storms aggravate. Cold also aggravates. Rhus pains is first a stiffness and soreness. There are also tearing pains, drawing, paralyzed sensations and even stitches. The sudden pain in the back known as "crick" is met well with Rhus. Rhus has an especial affinity for the deep muscles of the back. It is perhaps the most often indicated of any remedy in lumbago. It is also a remedy for the effects of overexertion such as sprains, wrenches. The rheumatism of Rhus may appear in any part of the body; the lower extremities seem to have suffered most in the provers. The great keynotes of Rhus are the following:

1. Relief from continued motion; the lumbago, however, being sometimes worse from motion.

2. The stiffness and soreness.

3. The aggravation when first beginning to move.

4. The aggravation from damp weather and cold. Cold air is not tolerated; it seems to make the skin painful.

5. The relief of all the symptoms by warmth.

Bryonia 6C to 30C -   The rheumatism of Bryonia attacks the joints themselves, producing articular rheumatism, and it also inflames the muscle tissue, causing muscular rheumatism. The muscles are sores and swollen, and the joints are violently inflamed, red, swollen, shiny, and very hot. The pains are sharp, stitching or cutting in character, and the great feature of the drug should always be present, namely the aggravation from the slightest motion. Touch and pressure also aggravate.

Causticum 6C to 30C - This remedy resembles Rhus quite closely in many respects. The following are some of the differences: Causticum - The restlessness of this remedy occurs only at night. Rheumatism caused by dry, cold frosty air. Pains impel constant motion, which does not relieve. Rhus - Restlessness all the time. Rheumatism from damp wet weather. Motion relieves the patient temporarily. The symptoms calling for Causticum are a stiffness of the joints. The tendons seem shortened and the limbs are drawn out of shape. It is a sort of rheumatoid arthritis. As with Rhus, there is relief from warmth. There are drawing muscular pains and soreness of the parts of which the patient lies. It has been found useful in rheumatism about the articulations of the jaw. There is much weakness and trembling with Causticum.

Ledum 6C to 30C - Ledum is one of our best remedies for rheumatism and gout, especially the latter. The great symptom which has always been regarded as the distinctive characteristic is the direction the pains take, namely, going from below upwards. Ledum seems to have a predilection for the smaller joints. Nodes form in them and the pains travel up the limbs. The pains are made worse from the warmth of the bed. The effusion into the joints is scanty and it soon hardens and forms the nodosities. Ledum causes acute, tearing pains in the joints; weakness of the limbs and numbness and coldness of the surface. Ledum may be thus summed up:

1. Upward extension of the pains.
2. Tendency to the formation of nodes in the small joints.
3. Aggravation by the warmth of the bed.
4. Aggravation by motion.

Pulsatilla 6C to 30C - Pulsatilla is usually brought to mind when there is a tendency for the rheumatism to shift about, wandering rheumatic pains being one of its red strings. Other characteristics of the Pulsatilla rheumatism are the aggravation from warmth, aggravation in the evening, and the relief from cold. The knee, ankle and tarsal joints are the most usual seat of the trouble when Pulsatilla is indicated. There is too a restlessness with the remedy, the pains are so severe that the patient is compelled to move, and slow, easy motion relieves. The joints are swollen and the pains are sharp and stinging, with a feeling of subcutaneous ulceration.

Kalmia 6C to 30C - Kalmia is another of the remedies which have wandering rheumatic pains, and it is especially useful in rheumatism affecting the chest, or when rheumatism or gout shifts from the joints to the heart, driven there perhaps by external applications. It also has tearing pains in the legs, without swelling, without fever, but with great weakness. The pains about the chest in Kalmia cases shoot down into the stomach and abdomen. The muscles of the neck are sore and the back is lames. The rheumatic pains are mostly in the upper parts of the arms and lower parts of the legs; and are worse when going to sleep. Inflammatory rheumatism, shifting from joint to joint, with tendency to attack the heart, high fever, excruciating pains, which, of course, are made worse by motion, will be benefited by Kalmia.

Cimicifuga 6C to 30C - Cimicifuga is a rheumatic remedy; its chief symptom is great aching in the muscles, and this right in the fleshy part of the muscles, the belly of the muscles rather than the extremities. It is also prone to occur in the large muscles of the trunk rather than the small muscles of the extremities, here resembling Nux vomica. Rheumatism in the muscles, coming on suddenly and of great severity, worse at night and in wet and windy weather will find its remedy in Cimicifuga. In Cimicifuga there is great restlessness, but motion aggravates.

Colchicum 6C to 30C - Although usually thought of in gout Colchicum is no mean remedy in rheumatism. It has a special affinity for fibrous tissues, tendons, aponeuroses, ligaments, and periosteum. It has also shifting rheumatism. The pains are worse in the evening; the slightest motion aggravates; the patient is irritable; the pain seems unbearable. Sometimes it is useful when the rheumatism attacks the chest, with pains about the heart and a sensation as if the heart were squeezed by a tight bandage. There is great evening aggravation; the joints are swollen and dark red. Colchicum is especially useful for rheumatic affections in debilitated persons those who are weak-weakness being the characteristic. It is a remedy too, for the smaller joints. Colchicum is rarely indicated early in rheumatism but later when the patient is weak and exhausted it may do good work.

Sanguinaria 6C to 30C - Sanguinaria inflames muscular tissue, giving a picture of acute muscular rheumatism. The muscles are sore and stiff, with flying erratic pains in them or stitching. The muscles of the back and neck are especially affected by it. The chief field of usefulness of the remedy seems to be in rheumatism affecting the right deltoid muscle. It is described as a rheumatic pain in the right arm and shoulder, worse at night or on turning in bed. It is so severe that the patient cannot raise the arm.

Phytolacca 6C to 30C - It is particularly useful in pains below the elbows and knees. There is stiffness and lameness of the muscles; the pains seem to fly about, are worse at night and are especially aggravated by damp weather. Rheumatic affections of the sheaths of the nerves; periosteal rheumatism or rheumatism of the fibrous tissues often is benefited by Phytolacca. Rheumatism of the shoulder and arms may call for this remedy. It cured a case of right deltoid rheumatism of twenty-seven years standing.

Guaiacum 6C to 30C - Guaiacum is a remedy with many rheumatic symptoms. It is in the chronic forms of articular rheumatism where the joints are distorted with concretions that it will do the most good, given earlier it will prevent the formation of these concretions. It is good remedy with which to follow Causticum. Symptoms will be contraction tendons, which draw the limb out of shape, worse on any motion. We have already seen a number of remedies having these deposits in the joints, but none having these contractions. Stiffness and soreness of the joints and soreness of the muscles are also present.

Gout - Metabolic Arthritis

Gout comes from the buildup of uric acid, but more from the supersaturated body fluids of uric acid that gravity pulls down to the peripheral joints and especially the big toe, which then crystalizes in and about the joints forming needle shaped crystals. Uric acid is made from the breakdown of the purine bases that compose of the genetic material of DNA. As cells die they release DNA which has purine bases that break down to uric acid. Add to that a high diet of protein loaded with DNA and acids from sugar etc we start to get a body overloaded with acid. If this is just beginning it would be a good idea to get a kidney function test as this is the organ whose main function is to get rid of all the acids. For about 10% of people there could be an added genetic problem which could be the cause so a thorough investigation is needed. Only 1 in 20 cases of hyperuricemia turn into Gout. Attacks of Gout are caused by the body's inflammatory response to the uric acid crystals in the joints. Acute attacks appear without warning with a rapid onset of severe joint pain, swelling and redness. They often begin at night after alcoholic beverages or high purine foods (anchovies, asparagus, crab, fish roe, herring, kidney, liver, meat gravies and broth, mushrooms, mussels, peas, beans and sardines). In 90% of early episodes only a single joint is involved usually the big toe. Latter the foot, heel, ankle, knee, hands, wrists and elbows can become involved. Attacks can last a few days to a few weeks. In about 10% of people they never have an attack again while with most there is usually a relapse in a year. Untreated cases can turn chronic and spread to other joints and there can be a buildup of uric acid in the skin behind the elbow on the wrist and on the ears, they are called tophi. High uric acid levels can eventually lead to kidney failure. **Cause** - The main type of Gout is genetic. It is a genetic defect in the enzymes that break down purine. Other causes can be a high acid diet and kidney failure. **Nutrition and Diet** - High acid diets are the cause of most diseases so we have to go back and study the Acid and Alkaline diet. Doing this can also show you just how far you are in the acid lane and what to do about it, and if you have Gout you are in the extreme of the acid lane and will probably have to focus on this diet for the rest of your life or wear out your kidneys. A high water intake is also needed as to dilute the acid in the system and to make it easier to flush out.

Also as mentioned before high purine foods should be removed from the diet and really cut back on protein especially meats and concentrate on the light proteins such as cheese milk and eggs. You may also have to lose some weight. **Treatment -** Main medical treatment is with the drug Zyloprim allopurionol which inhibits the xanthine oxidase enzyme which prevents the formation of uric acid and Gout. **Herbal Treatment -** With everything in this condition at its nastiest and severe levels there is not much we can do except concentrate on the cause which is massive acid build up. Here we are just going to work with diuretics so as to flush the acids out of the body, so you have to up your water intake so we have fluid to work with that will first dilute the acids which our diuretics will then flush through the kidneys to remove the acids and other wastes. Look back to Osteoarthritis and Rheumatism and choose two diuretics out of the choice of Celery Seed, Nettles, Ginger, Meadowsweet and Pansy, make it the one most suited to you. To this we are going to add one of Herbalism's best and safest diuretics which is Dandelion Leaf. Diuretics during their work tend to take potassium out of the body as well which is not good as the body uses potassium and salt as the main water or fluid balancers. You all know salt raises blood pressure because it sucks water into the blood well potassium sucks water into the cells so between Salt and Potassium water balance is maintained in the body. Dandelion Leaf is loaded with potassium so it puts back what most diuretics take out. As the pain is severe in this condition I shall leave it to your Doctor to supply a strong pain killer and here we will just concentrate on taking out the cause and getting your diet right so you don't have to go through this again. The only thing I would suggest is the formula below in powder form which is used by lots of athletes and horses to heal joint injuries fast which I have given to many people and had the feedback that it was really good for my Gout. This will work a little bit as a pain killer but what I am really using it for is to minimize the damage and repair it faster. This should be fairly easy to find as lots of people use it now for arthritis.

Glucosamine Sulphate, Chondroitin Sulphate and (MSM) Formula

Glucosamine Sulphate - Has many biological functions among which is its role as a stimulant and precursor to the proteins that form cartilage. As we age our ability to produce GS decreases and causes the cartilage to lose its water holding capability causing the cartilage to becomes dry and ineffective as a shock absorber, leading to pain. GS normalizes cartilage metabolism and prevents cartilage degradation. Stimulates the biosynthesis of the key structural components of cartilage (mucopolysaccharides) that are essential for healthy joint function and repair. Mucopolysaccharides also allow the cartilage to hold water which in turn acts as a shock absorber. GS also acts as a mild anti-inflammatory and combines with **Chondroitin** for effective joint repair and helps relieve the pain and inflammation of arthritis and joint injuries. Beneficial to athletes affected by cartilage or joint problems and halts cartilage destruction and encourages the regeneration of new cartilage.

Chondroitin Sulphate - Occurs naturally in the cartilage where it participates in the matrix structure. CS protects cartilage from degradation by inhibiting elastase which is the enzyme responsible for the degradation of cartilage and increases the synthesis of proteoglycans which is a key structural component of cartilage. Together with GS, CS has been found to increase hyaluronate concentration and viscosity of synovial fluid increasing lubrication within the joints. Like GS, CS exerts only a mild anti-inflammatory action and for this reason both are usually given together with anti-inflammatory nutrients such as MSM and bioflavonoids in order to obtain faster pain relief. Vitamins C, E, B3, B5, and B6 are also valuable adjuncts to supplementation with GS and CS.

Methyl Sulfonyl Methane (MSM) - Is a naturally occurring source of organic Sulphur. The concentration of Sulphur in arthritic cartilage has been shown to be about one third the level of normal cartilage. Other beneficial effects of MSM are due to its ability to reduce inflammation and to inhibit pain impulses along nerve fibers. Can be of benefit in conditions of bursitis, tendonitis, tennis elbow and RSI. As we age the levels of MSM in the body decrease.

Homoeopathic Treatment - **Choose the remedy that suits you and you should be able to find a write up of that remedy in Osteoarthritis or Rheumatism.**

GOUT

By W.A. Dewey

Dewey gives the common homeopathic remedies for the treatment of Gout in an easy question-answer format. …

When is Colchicum indicated in gout?
Where the swelling is red or pale, with extreme tenderness to touch and tendency to shift about from joint to joint; pains are worse in. the evening and from the slightest motion; metastasis of gout to heart, with cutting pains about heart and oppression.

Give indications for Ammonium phosphoricum in Gout.
Constitutional gout with nodes and concretions in the joints chronic cases where these concretions of` Urate of Soda deform the joints.

What are the symptoms calling for arnica in Gout?
Extreme soreness.
What of the use of Ledum?
Pains worse from the warmth of the bed; drawing pains in joints scanty effusion, which tends to harden into nodosities.
How does Bryonia compare?
Ledum produces a scanty effusion, which tends to harden into nodosities, while Bryonia tends to a copious effusion.
Give some other remedies having nodular swellings in the joints.
Calcarea carb, Benzoic acid, Lycopodium, Lithium carb and Antimonium crud.
Give symptoms of Guaiacum in Gout.
Concretions of the joints. 'gouty inflammation of the knee with abscess. Contractions of muscles.

Osteoporosis

This disorder is characterized by a slow and progressive thinning and loss of the calcium content of the bones along with other minerals. Although the process actually begins in the fourth decade in both sexes it is accelerated in women after menopause. We all know the nasty things that can happen like hip fracture etc etc so I won't go into details. Early symptoms are those of calcium deficiency which are excessive nervousness, muscle twitching, nocturnal cramps, high blood pressure and dull bone pain in the long bones of limbs and not confined to any special area. The problem is more common in women where it causes spinal pain and stooped posture which is the end result of osteoporosis. There is dull aching which is sharp and episodic with stooped posture and respiratory distress, by then it is too late. Always remember prevention is much easier than cure. Consider getting a bone density test for females at 55 and males at 60 years of age and if you get good results test again every 5 years. Prevention is the best way to go.

High Risk Factors for Osteoporosis
1. A diet high in animal protein
2. Women who are light boned.
3. People with low bone density scared to exercise.

4.   People who have been on lots of punishing diets.
5.   Women who smoke as this brings on menopause earlier.
6.   Women who have a genetic predisposition to it ie mother has it.
7.   Poor unbalanced diet especially those high in acid.
8.   Caffeine and alcohol encourage the excretion of calcium.
9.   Excessive salt intake.
10. Drugs - Cortisone, thyroxine, tamoxifen, diuretics and antacids.
11. Total hysterectomies including removal of their ovaries.
12. Being underweight.
13. Poor absorption of nutrients by the digestive system.
14. Being bed ridden or an invalid with no exercise.

Nutrition for Osteoporosis

Calcium supplements are often poorly absorbed especially inorganic sources such as dolomite. Calcium should be combined with magnesium in the ratio of 2 to 1. A supplement should ideally contain other minerals and vitamins needed in the right proportions. Calcium taken alone depletes zinc and iron. Try a supplement that goes something like this 1000mg calcium, 500mg magnesium, 10mg zinc, 3mg boron and a bit of Vitamin D. Take with it about 1000mg of vitamin C daily. Always try to get Calcium made from animal bones as we know these have been absorbed by something living so we have a good chance of absorbing it to. Even better try to get your calcium and minerals naturally from the diet, the only problem here is that only about 20 to 40% of calcium is absorbed and this gets worse with age. Vitamin D is needed for the absorption of calcium and for the body to make vitamin D it needs exposure to sunlight so make sure you get a bit of sun every day, go for a walk. Milk and other dairy products are not necessarily the best sources for natural calcium. Milk is low in magnesium which is needed to assimilate calcium and there are other foods that are higher. The table below suggests some other sources.

Boron - Boron is required for strong bones and the full absorption of calcium. Sources are apples, pears, grapes, dates, raisins, peaches, soybeans, almonds, hazelnuts, peanuts and honey. As a micro nutrient the dose is small about 1 to 2mg a day so a good dose is 2 apples and 3 and a half ounces of peanuts.

Calcium Rich Foods	
Kelp (sea weed) per 100 grams	1093mg
Blackstrap molasses per 100 grams	579mg
Sardines per 100 grams	550mg
Dried figs per 100 grams	280mg
Almonds per 100 grams	250mg
Watercress per 100 grams	220mg
Sunflower seeds per 100 grams	100mg
Tofu per 100 grams	128mg
Comparison With Dairy Foods	
Cow's milk per 100mls	120mg
Cheddar Cheese per 50 grams	400mg
Yoghurt per 100 grams	180mg

Herbal Treatment - Treat as for malabsorption problems and take herbs that activate calcium absorption and supply easily assimilated Calcium eg Comfrey, Irish Moss, Slippery Elm and Fenugreek which is virtually a multivitamin in its own right. Also consider using the Cell Salts Calc Phos 6X (Tissue Salts) and if you like the Tissue Salts add Mag Phos 6X as well with any formulation you like as it will add to the assimilation. Comfrey poultices and cream can be used on the affected areas. Comfrey and Arnica cream can be mixed together as the Arnica cream can help if the area feels bruised and sore but never use Arnica close or on an open wound.

Calcium Assimilation Formula - These herbs help in the absorption of calcium rather than being a rich source, they are mucilage and they balance the digestion so calcium supplements can be absorbed better by cleansing the bowel and the blood, freeing the absorption sites, they also supply some bioavailable calcium. Bitter saponins assist absorption of calcium while bitter diuretics increase elimination of wastes via the urinary system. Nutritive herbs provide rich sources of manganese essential for the absorption of calcium and provide other cofactors such as phosphorus and Vit D needed for calcium absorption. These are the herbs that are used in the old formulas so I am not going to change them much as it is also about the mechanics of the formula as well as the herbs. (Warning Comfrey is illegal to use internally in Australia even as a small part of a formula. External use only in Australia. Please ask the AMA for an explanation as I will not be capable of controlling my language). Below is a good soothing formula for those with tummy problems. Take you calcium tablet 20 minutes after the formula and if it is a compressed powder type of tablet chew it up and wash it down with a bit of milk as this will make the pill semi digested before it goes to digestion. Remember that the longer and further you can spread out the tablet along the 30 feet of small intestine the more the body can absorb.

Calcium Formula for Unhappy Tummies

Comfrey 20 to 30%

Marshmallow 20 to 30

Slippery elm 10 to 20

Irish moss 10 to 20

These are the mucilage herbs and they reduce bowel transit time, regulate colonic bacteria, absorb toxins from the bowel (Especially Slippery Elm) and are demulcent which means they will soothe the inflamed areas as they travel.

Highest plant sources of

Calcium - Valerian, buchu leaves, white oak bark, kelp, nettle, Senna, cramp bark, barberry, horsetail, Irish moss.

Manganese - Irish moss, oatstraw, licorice, kelp, bladderwrack, nettle, senna, peppermint leaves, white willow, pennyroyal, burdock root, chick weed.

Phosphorus - Cabbage herb, bilberry, pumpkin seeds, soyabeans, peppermint leaves, yellow dock root, milk thistle, buchu leaves, fennel, mulien, hops, calamus, garlic, meadowsweet.

K Campion Formula

Horsetail 6 parts

Comfrey 4 parts

Nettle 3 parts

Kelp 1 part

Meadowsweet 1 part

Finely powdered 2 x size O capsules with each meal.

Heinerman - Calcium Supplement.
Comfrey root - calcium, phosphorous
Horsetail - calcium, silicon
Oatstraw
Lobelia
4 to 6 capsules a day.
Indicated for - arthritis, rheumatism, osteoporosis, pregnancy, lactation, tooth decay, numbness of arm and leg, nervousness, menstrual cramps, menopausal problems, hormone balance (parathyroid), blood clotting, growth, insomnia, obesity.

Vitamin D
Is produced in the skin with the help of sunshine or UV light. This is the first stage, then from here it is transported to the liver where it is changed again and from there it goes to the third and final change which takes place in the kidney. The action of parathyroid hormone is to activate the kidneys. From here the active form of vit D goes to the intestinal epithelium to help absorb calcium, to do this the body must also have sufficient Vit A.
Oestrogen in females has a marked effect on the activation of the kidneys. In premenopausal women from the age of 35 on there is decreased calcium in bones, increased levels of parathormone and decreased calcium balance. Normal daily requirement of calcium is 800 to 1200 mgs.
Factors that increase requirement are
Heavy exercise
High protein diet
Vegetarian diet
If calcium intake is not sufficient it leads to release of parathormone which takes the calcium from the bones.
Sources - Sunshine and herbs – alfalfa, nettles, watercress.
Foods - wheat germ, fish liver oils, egg yolk.
Vit D is necessary for healthy bones and teeth, proper assimilation and for the body to balance calcium and phosphorous.

Homoeopathic Treatment for Osteoporosis

Calcaria Phos 6X – Is an excellent remedy for osteoporosis and is also known as one of the main Tissue Salts (Calc Phos 6C). Delicate and easily breakable bones. This will promote the absorption of calcium from the food that the patient takes. The bones of the extremities are also weak and fragile. Stools green, undigested and offensive. Good to take for fractures or any injury to the bone. No appetite, it is a bone builder and creates new blood cells. It gives general tone to the entire organism. Promotes the absorption of calcium.

Calcaria Iod 6C – Should be thought of when there is deficiency of muscles and fat in addition to deficiency of bones. Unhealthy condition of glands is always present when this remedy is indicated.

Lumbago

Lumbago these days is more a generic term that refers to pain in the lower back region or lumber region. Lots of people have this at one time or another especially those over 50. You worry here when it does not go away. **Symptoms** - It's important to recognize the basic signs that could suggest lumbago. Pain that's located in the lumbar area of the spine is the primary symptom. Typically, this pain includes lower back stiffness, muscle tension and aches and pains. In the worst cases, mobility can be compromised. Movement may be restricted such as when you try to bend over or lean backwards. If the pain is in the butt and radiates down the leg and feels nervy then you may have sciatica which is a nerve problem. Sometimes the cause of lumbago is hard to pinpoint even after lots of medical tests. Lumbago can be caused from several factors but the main reason is the overuse of the lower back, a sudden lifting of a heavy load, repetitive or excessive movement of the lower back, a slipped or herniated disc, compression of a spinal nerve, Osteoarthritis and maybe Rheumatism may also be the cause. **Treatment** - Glucosamine Sulphate, Chondroitin Sulphate and (MSM) Formula as seen in Gout is where I usually start. As mentioned this can be found in a powdered formula that you mix with water that allows you to get maximum absorption of the supplement and usually covers most sprains and strains and if it doesn't it will protect and ease the pain while you are waiting for help and start the repair. **Herbal Treatment** - Provide pain relief and improve circulation by massaging with a liniment of something like Winter Green oil, St John's Wort oil, Arnica oil with a teaspoon full of cayenne in carrier oil. Never use on broken skin or close to a wound. Herbs to promote healing of spinal discs and improve their lubrication when deteriorated, fused, slipped or ruptured are comfrey, fenugreek, marshmallow, Irish moss and slippery elm. Comfrey and fenugreek help replace the soft pulpy cushion between the discs.

Homoeopathic Treatment for Lumbago

Arnica 6C - For the shock and bruised sore pains. Arnica cream can also be applied as long as the skin is not broken.

Bellis Perennis 6C - Deeper acting then Arnica, intense soreness of the muscles, where swellings and lumps remain after the injury.

Ledum 6C - Injuries where the swollen part is cold or numb, sometimes looks purple and puffy, feels better for cold applications.

Ruta 6C - If the bones inside or near the joint feel bruised.

Bone Injuries and Fractures

The main remedy here is Comfrey or to use its old fashioned name knitbone. This is good to use on the injured area when the cast is removed as it will help to strengthen the mend. For areas that cannot have casts on or for fine fractures Comfrey is ideal and will speed up the healing process. Comfrey has a chemical in it that speeds up cell division, it is also astringent and mucilage which gives it soothing and protecting qualities and has been used for hundreds of years in the healing of bones and wounds. I always add Calc Phos 6X to people taking Comfrey for fractures and also add a good Calcium Supplement like the one mentioned in Osteoporosis. As mentioned before it is illegal to use Comfrey internally in Australia but for the rest of the world I have made a write-up on the herb by many authors and will leave it to you to make your own decisions. **Herbal Treatment** - Apply cream to affected area regularly, if you grow comfrey in your garden you can make a poultice out of the leaves and apply it to the affected area.

Comfrey

Symphytum officinalis

Actions - Demulcent, astringent, healing, expectorant, vulnerary, cell proliferant, bone healer.

Once widely cultivated as a fodder plant, sheep and cows eat it greedily so the plant was easily available to local populations who used it as a natural remedy especially in bone fractures. The impressive wound healing powers of comfrey are partially due to allantoin which stimulates cell proliferation and speeds the healing process inside and out. Also used in the treatment of diarrhoea, dysentery and shallow G.I. ulcers. These conditions respond to the demulcent, vulnerary, astringent and anti-inflammatory properties of the plant. The astringent action reduces haemorrhage associated with ulcers and colitis. Bronchial irritation and irritated coughs with hemoptysis (spitting blood) respond well. Comfrey tablets were even standard issue in World War II First Aid packs for the British as so widely known was the ability of this herb to speed up the healing of bones and wounds. It is very important to make sure that wounds are completely clean before applying Comfrey – this is because the skin can regrow so fast that it can trap any debris left in the wound, also bear in mind that the surface of the wound may heal and close faster than the deeper parts of the wound. When used in wounds ensure that they are well cleaned and no foreign bodies are left inside as the skin can regrow so fast that it can trap debris left in the wound. Good for chronic varicose ulcers. Its old name is knit bone and that describes well what it does. Comfrey also guards against scar tissue from developing incorrectly. Used for all internal hemorrhages including uterine, reunion of wound and fractures, internal ulcers, ruptures, pulmonary problems, bronchitis, irritable cough, ulcerative colitis, skin ulcers and varicose veins. Comfrey is typically used to make compresses, poultices, ointments and salves to be applied topically. **Constituents** - Alkaloid (pyrrolizidine) (root only), mucilage, gum, tannin, silicic acid, phenolic acid (caffeic, rosmarinic, chlorogenic), allantoin, asparagine, choline, chlorophyll, Ca, K+, P, trace minerals, vitamins A and C. **Caution -** Short-term dosing only. 2

to 3 weeks on and 3 weeks off. **Precautions** - If taking Comfrey internally it is best done on the advice of a Herbal Practitioner due to the potential effects of pyrrolizidine alkaloids on the liver. Pregnant and nursing mothers should not use Comfrey. **Dose – Source from a Professional.** Tincture - 2 to 4mls 3 times daily. Decoction – 1 to 3 teaspoons full of dried herb into cup of boiling water for 10 to 15 minutes. Used as Ointment, Cream, Lotion, Fomentation, Compresses, Poultices, Washes, Baths.

Homoeopathic Treatment for Fractures

Follow normal first aid procedures, if the bone is obviously broken it is best to call an ambulance. If you do have to move the patient make sure the injured limb is supported or a sharp piece of bone may cut an internal artery. Most bone injuries need x-rays to determine the extent of the damage.

Arnica 6C - Can be given straight away for the shock and will help ease the pain from the bruising and swelling.

Ledum 6C - Take after Arnica 4 hourly or 3 times a day to assist in the absorption of the extravasation of blood after a fracture so as to reduce the swelling which may take up to 3 to 4 days. (Helps to absorb the internal bleeding after a fracture)

After the bones have been set properly use these two remedies

CalcPhos 6X - Helps in nutrition especially of the bones and promotes the knitting together of the bones. Helps fractures heal much faster. Can be used in alternation with Symphytum 6C.

Symphytum 6C - More commonly known as Comfrey or knitbone or bone set. The name says it all. Promotes fast healing of bones, use with Calc Phos 6X. Take both 3 times daily till recovered.

Muscle Cramps

Muscle cramps are sudden involuntary contractions that occur in various muscles. These contractions are often painful and can affect different muscle groups. Commonly affected muscles are those in the back of your lower leg, the back of your thigh, and the front of your thigh. You can also experience cramps in your abdominal wall, arms, hands, feet and toes. The intense pain of a cramp can awaken you at night especially in the calf. **Symptoms -** Sudden sharp twitching pain, lasting from a few seconds to 15 minutes is the most common symptom of a muscle cramp. In some cases a bulging lump of muscle tissue beneath the skin can accompany a cramp which can sometimes be rubbed and massaged back into place. **Causes -** The cause usually lies in the nervous system or the nutritional status of the person. Make sure that you drink enough liquid to avoid dehydration. Your body loses more water when physically active or you live in a hot area in summer, so increase your liquid intake when you exercise or the temperature is hotter than normal. People who are older generally don't have as much muscle mass and may stress muscles more easily leading to cramping. People living with diabetes, liver disorders, nerve compression, and thyroid disorders may experience muscle cramps. Some cramps result from overused or tired muscles usually while you're exercising. Other causes are dehydration, old injuries and poor nutrition especially being low in calcium, potassium, sodium and magnesium. Another cause is low blood supply to the area which is more common in the legs, I see this one fairly frequently as I do Iridology and in the eye it shows up as a white ring around the edge of the color of your eye and is known as a Sodium or Calcium Ring and it means blood supply is decreased through the main thigh and neck arteries. **Herbal Treatment -** For a very simple and effective treatment make a Chamomile tea (this may work by itself) and take a good calcium supplement as mentioned in Osteoporosis but chew the supplement to powder first and wash it down with the tea or you could powder the supplement and put it in the tea. Old tummies are not the best at digestion and we want something that works and can give us a yes or no answer fast. The main remedy for cramping is Cramp Bark which lives up to its name. Generally we use it with Prickly Ash which is a peripheral circulation stimulant which means it gets blood into the arms and legs and its also antispasmodic and a pain killer so it will be adding these actions to the Cramp Bark which is below. Use a good Calcium formula with these two remedies along with the Tissue Salts mentioned in the Homoeopathic section especially Mag Phos 6X which can usually do the job all by itself.

Cramp Bark

Viburnum opulus

Actions - Nervine, sedative, astringent, antispasmodic, tonic, emmenagogue, dysmenorrhea, nervous system relaxant, anti-asthmatic, hypotensive, peripheral vasodilator, muscle relaxant.

As the name suggests this herb relaxes muscular tension and spasms. It has two main areas of use with the first being muscular cramps and the second in ovarian and uterine muscle problems. Cramp Bark relaxes the uterus and relieves spasms and cramps and was used in the past to help prevent miscarriages. The anti-spasmodic compounds in Cramp Bark work on all other types of cramps in the body including bronchial, gastrointestinal, genitourinary and skeletal muscle spasms. As a skeletal muscle relaxant, it is particularly effective for leg cramps. Its astringent action gives it a role in the treatment of excessive blood loss in periods and especially bleeding associated with the menopause. With spasms consider adding a supplement of magnesium as this could be deficient. Restores the sympathetic and parasympathetic nervous systems balance in voluntary and involuntary muscle spasms of the autonomic nervous system. Cramp Barks peripheral vasodilator action helps restore the blood flow to the arms and legs and helps to supply the magnesium that is needed. Cramp Bark is also rich in valerenic acid which is named from the sedative herb Valerian which was later used in the making of Valium. **Part Used** - Dried cortex (bark). **Combinations -** For the relief of cramp it may be combined with Prickly Ash and if severe Wild Yam. For severe leg cramps which won't go away add Ginkgo Biloba as it will open up the main arteries in the legs. For uterine and ovarian pains or threatened miscarriage it may be used with Black Haw and Valerian. **Precautions -** Do not use Cramp Bark if you have aspirin sensitivity. Not recommended for those on blood thinning medications. **Doses** - Tincture 4 to 8mls three times a day, for tea 2 teaspoonful's of the dried bark 3 times a day.

Homoeopathic Treatment for Muscle Cramps

Tissue Salts - Mag Phos 6X, Calc Phos 6X, Kali Phos 6X. **Mag Phos 6X** is the main one here that my father used to use as soon as he stopped hoping around the bed he would add 2 to 3 tablets in half a glass of warm water and get relief in 10 to 15 minutes.

Fibromyalgia

Fibromyalgia is a chronic condition characterized by pain in the muscles, ligaments, and tendons along with fatigue and there can also be multiple tender points or spots in the body. This is one of the hardest diseases to deal with for both the patient and their Doctor and all the lab tests will not help as they just don't know what it is, or the cause. The disease seems to pick on women far more than men and also tends to coexist with sleep disorders, anxiety, depression, and irritable bowel syndrome and increased sensitivity to pain due to a decreased pain threshold along with a kind of chronic fatigue. Your first impression is that it is a kind of autoimmune disease. There is evidence that people with the condition may be more sensitive to pain because something is wrong with the body's usual pain perception processes. The disease can make life a misery but it is not degenerative or life-threatening. **Symptoms** – Almost all cases ache all over and they may also have tender points or areas that can hurt even from a gentle prod of a finger. Other symptoms can be depression and or anxiety, memory lapses and or difficulty in concentrating, trouble sleeping, a type of chronic fatigue, heightened sensitivity to noises, bright lights or smells. Irritable bowel syndrome (IBS) and or Restless legs syndrome (RLS) seem also to be involved in this disease. Other symptoms are skin sensitivity, dizziness, headaches, numbness, and tingling in hands, arms, and legs. I will leave it there as with this disease you could go on forever as it's very confusing and always hurts my brain. **Treatment** – With a disease as complex as this with no obvious cure, that goes on for a long time and ruins your quality of life, your main herbs have to be from the Adaptogens as I doubt you could give any quality of life or hope without using a long term herb for chronic conditions. Here we have to treat the worst of the patient's conditions in the order they wish to give them some quality of life again and some hope. This disease may be genetic so start by asking has anyone else in your family had this condition. We will start with an example patient having chronic pain all over and being depressed and anxious and thinking about their future and how they are going to carry on. Hopefully the adaptogens I am intending to use will help them function as well as possible on a daily basis. The first adaptogen that we will use first is called Shizandra which is the herb I use to fix up damaged nerves and we will use it for a week by itself to see what happens. The main reason I am starting here is that the specific drug for this disease which the doctors use is called Pregabalin, which is used for damaged nerves. After the week and depending on the results we will start treatment for the chronic pain, which I hope has been reduced, and depression and anxiety. After this I will keep adding with different scenarios.

Schisandra

Actions – Adaptogen, immune stimulant, anti-inflammatory, liver and kidney tonic, restorative, nervous system tonic, mild anti-depressant, anti-anxiety and anti-stress, adrenal tonic, antioxidant, astringent, anti-tussive, lung tonic, regulates blood pressure, anti-cholesterol, sedative.

Of great use as a general liver protector that works well in the treatment of hepatitis. It is a liver detoxifier and works to deactivate free radicals that attack liver cells. Being extremely high in powerful antioxidants Schisandra helps to fight against free radical damage, thus lowering inflammatory responses. Can help in the nervous system by increasing the nervous reflex response and can also help in anxiety, depression, neurosis and stress. Promotes vitality and increases memory along with cognitive functions while providing resistance to stress. Is a powerful anti-anxiety herb lowering stress levels and enhancing mental performance. Because of its adaptogenic qualities it specifically reduces both mental and physical stress, exerting a normalising effect on the whole body. Schisandra reduces cortisol levels in the body (the stress hormone) and is effective in controlling changes in serotonin and adrenaline caused by stress. The herb is also considered a lung tonic because it helps the body to better utilize oxygen. Because Schisandra is high in powerful antioxidants it lowers the inflammatory responses, which in turn positively affects, tones and strengthens the immune system along with increasing physical performance and endurance and promotes recovery after surgery. Schisandra has long been used in the traditional medicines of China and Russia for a wide variety of ailments. As far back as 2697 BCE Schisandra was listed in the Yellow Emperor's Study of Inner Medicine, an encyclopaedia of healing plants. **Precautions** - Mild side effects may include indigestion, nausea, headaches and skin rash. Schisandra may promote contractions of the uterine muscles and thus should not be used by pregnant women. **Contraindications** - Avoid in fever. **Part Used** - Fruit (berries). **Dose** – Tincture 3 mls up to 3 times daily. Infusions - 1 to 2 tea spoons full to cup of boiling water 3 up to 3 times daily. Can also be found in powder and tablet form.

Schisandra is my kind of clearing the deck herb which should be of great help in the first week as you should have noted in reading it through. This herb is my tool for repairing damaged nerves and I use it mainly in people who have had strokes with an example being someone having problems with their arms which may lack strength, or the hand keeps dropping things. There can also be shooting pains. As this is a long lasting disease Schisandras week could give us valuable clues for the future treatment of the condition. Withania is our next main herb and another adaptogen which means they try to adapt you to your condition giving you more energy, strength and endurance. Adaptogens are usually given in diseases that are going to be long and drawn out such as cancers. This herb happily works together with Shisandra along with being a female friendly herb as in the past it was used to prevent miscarriages and to help women to the full term of their pregnancy and Fibromyalgia is known to pick on women more than men.

Withania

(Ashwagandha)

Actions - Adaptogen, analgesic, anti-tumor, hormone regulator, pregnancy tonic, rejuvinative, anti-inflammatory, sedative, anti-anemic.

Used to restore health to the nervous system and eases stress and mental exhaustion. Good for debility, nervous exhaustion especially due to stress and chronic diseases especially those marked by inflammation. Retards various aspects of the aging process and increases stamina. Promotes mental clarity and improves memory and stamina. **Relieves pain by lowering serotonin levels which contribute to the sensitivity of pain receptors in the body.** Tonic for the elderly and improves conditions associated with ageing. Promotes recovery after illness and during convalescence and has great use in various chronic diseases involving inflammation. Can aid bone degeneration, rheumatism, joint pain and neuralgias.

Dose - As on packet.

This is an ideal herb for Fibromyalgia with its painkilling and anti-inflammatory actions along with its serotonin adjustments. These two herbs cover a lot of the symptoms of this disease and should give you a good start in trying to restore your health and as they are both Adaptogens you could make them the foundation of your treatment adding other herbs if and when you need them. As you have now met your 2 new friends we shall carry on to Depression and Anxiety which can play a big part in this disease. I am starting with Depression first as one of our main herbs used for Depression is also an excellent painkiller in its own right as well as being just as good as some medical anti-depressants and is known and used for shooting pains down nerve pathways (shingles) and stabbing like pains. The herb is St John's Wort also known as Hypericum. This herb also has a strong anti-viral action and as no one knows the cause of Fibromyalgia if it's a virus then we are another step ahead.

Depression

Here we will deal mainly with simple depression. Depression is a mood disorder that causes persistent feelings of sadness and loss of interest that affects how you feel, think and behave and can lead to a variety of emotional and physical problems. Everyone gets sad and upset but depression lasts longer and interferes with your daily life. Depression can be mild, moderate, or severe. You can have a single episode of depression or depression that comes back or lasts a long time. Major Depression can last for 2 weeks but often it can go on for over 20 weeks. Next we have to look at the causes with a good example being the death of a loved spouse, that would really hurt. This example is known as Adjustment Disorder. Another example is Postpartum Disorder of mothers may have depression after giving birth. **Causes -** People with depression may have abnormal levels of brain chemicals called neurotransmitters, including serotonin, dopamine, and norepinephrine. These may contribute to having depression. Also it is beginning to look like depression could have a heredity cause as it seems to run in families but more research needs to be done. Nutrition is also another obvious cause so have a good look at the diet, especially think of the B Vitamins and then calcium and magnesium. More women than men seem to have depression but this may not be true as women are more open to doctors while men don't tell them much. **Symptoms** – With Fibromyalgia the onset could be different but carry on reading how depression normally comes on in case you can see some similarities. Depression often comes on very slowly so it can be hard to figure out what is happening and sometimes the individual doesn't even know it themselves until a close friend and family member starts pointing out the changes. Look out for continuous low mood or sadness, having low self-esteem, changes in appetite or weight, low sex drive, lack of energy, difficult to fall asleep at night or waking up very early in the morning, irritable and intolerant of others, no motivation or interest in things, avoiding contact with friends and taking part in fewer social activities, neglecting your hobbies and interests, difficulties in your home, work or family life, trouble concentrating. Also look at the Homoeopathic remedies as I have tried to write them as person pictures so as you read them you should be able to imagine that I am describing a person. **Diagnosis -** As depression does not usually go away on its own speak to your doctor so they can run tests to rule out other conditions such as thyroid problems. Most medications for depression take 2 to 4 weeks to start working and may take up to 12 weeks for their full effects to kick in. **Herbal Treatment** – Here we will start with **Oats** as it will do what's needed on the nutrition side. You need to find the least processed Oats (for making porridge) that you can, so go to a Health Shop and buy a big bag of them. Naturopaths will use Oats in the Tincture or Extract form as these take nearly everything out of the Oats that they want. Oats is used for nervous debility and exhaustion associated with depression and is commonly used with Skullcap which is our next herb. **Skullcap** relaxes states of nervous tension while generally helping the whole of the Central Nervous System and for hysterical states. Good for exhausted and depressed conditions. **Vervain** is another good and relaxing nerve tonic that can also ease depression and times of hysteria. Mind and body techniques, such as biofeedback, meditation, and Tai Chi, may help prevent or reduce symptoms of depression. Some types of meditation while not only relaxing, you kind of put a pattern on the brain, imagine that you learnt this meditation months ago before the depression and now that the depression has come on you decide to try it again. In some the brain will jump back into the familiar pattern and give relief to the depression. Think of it as formatting the hard drive.

Damiana

Turnera diffusa

Actions - Nerve tonic, antidepressant, laxative, urinary antiseptic, stomachic.

Strengthening remedy for the nervous system, tonic action on hormone system, for anxiety and depression especially with a sexual association, tonic to the male reproductive system for impotence, anxiety and neurosis. Tonic for the aged especially in senile decay. For males it is specially indicated for alleviating problems of achieving and maintaining erections. Damiana also works to relieve stress and anxiety related to fears of inadequate sexual performance. One of the active constituents of this herb is thymol which is a compound that is responsible for Damiana's life enhancing and stimulating effect on the mind and body. Used for mild to moderate depression, anxiety and nervous exhaustion. Its stimulating and restorative properties make it a valuable herb for anxiety and depression occurring together as can often happen as a result of long term stress. **Contraindications** – pregnancy. **Parts Used** – Leaves. **Dose** – Tincture 1 to 2 mls 3 times daily. Infusion 1 teaspoon full to cup of boiling water.

Hypericum

St John's Wort

Actions - Anti-inflammatory, astringent, anti-viral, anti-spasmodic, nervine, vulnerary, antibacterial and antidepressant. St John's Wort is perhaps the most studied herb for depression with literally thousands of studies and clinical trials performed to assess its usefulness as an antidepressant. Many studies have found the herb to be equally as effective as traditional antidepressants, but with fewer side effects in mild to moderately depressed patients. This is not meant to be used in major suicidal depression. Taken internally it has a sedative and pain reducing effect, which gives it a place in the treatment of neuralgia, anxiety, tension and general depression. Hyperforin which is a component of Hypericum can inhibit synaptosomal reuptake of serotonin, norepinephrine, and dopamine. It may take 2 to 4 weeks to notice clinical results when taken for depression. Useful in mild to moderate depression, anxiety, neuralgia and myalgia's and generally for pains shooting down nerve pathways. This herb is antiviral both internally and topically. **Contraindications -** Can interfere with MAOIs, SSRIs, narcotics and reserpine. Do not use St. John's Wort during pregnancy or lactation. **Caution -** Photosensitivity can occur in susceptible individuals. Fair-skinned individuals should take precautions when exposed to the sun and the elderly should use protective eyewear when exposed. **Part Used** – Aerial and flowering parts. **Dosage** – Tincture 2 to 4mls three times daily. Infusion – 1 to 2 teaspoonsful of herb infused into a cup of boiling water taken 3 times daily.

Homoeopathic Remedies for Depression

Ignatia 30C – Good for acute cases. Leading remedy for treating depression. Good for cases of acute depression that has just begun. Those who need it remain sad all the time and may have weeping spells. They also isolate themselves and avoid social engagements. They brood all the time lost in deep thought which makes them sad and worried. They may be very irritable. Depression in teenagers. Depression due to grief and worry. Depression that gets triggered by acute grief like the death of a loved one, broken relationships and disappointments in life. Is often best for sensitive people that tend to suppress disappointment or grief. They also do not want to appear vulnerable, defensive, temperamental, or guarded in the eyes of others. Some of the other symptoms may also include insomnia, headaches and abdominal cramps. Not wanting to cry or appear too vulnerable to others, they may seem guarded, defensive and moody. They may also burst out laughing or in to tears, for no apparent reason. Insomnia or excessive sleeping. A feeling of a lump in the throat and heaviness in the chest with frequent sighing or yawning are leading indications of this remedy.

Natrum Mur – 30C - Is used more to treat cases of chronic depression. It is suited to those who are very sensitive, accompanied by sporadic episodes of weeping. They remain absorbed in grief all the time and dwell on the unpleasant memories of the past. They don't like consolation, and it worsens the complaints. They have a tendency to get offended easily. Along with it, they don't have an interest in doing any sort of work. They will often hide inner feelings such as anger, fear of misfortune, grief, or affection. They are also responsible, reserved, guarded, and they seek solitude. Although they also seek sympathy, they can become angry if someone attempts to console them. Anxiety, brooding about past grievances, migraines, back pain, and insomnia can also be experienced when the person is depressed. A craving for salt and tiredness from sun exposure are other indications for this remedy. Other symptoms include migraines, insomnia, back pain, anxiety, and hopelessness.

Aurum Met 30C – For Hopelessness, Worthlessness and Suicidal Thoughts. A remedy for the workaholic with a tendency toward worthlessness, despair, and suicidal thoughts after a failure at work or in their personal life. An effective remedy for depression for patients who are very serious people, strongly focussed on work and achievement, who become depressed if they feel they have failed in some way. Nervous breakdown. Feel that they are worthless and of no value. They assume negative thoughts and the future seems dark to them. They feel that life is a burden, it's useless to live, and they long for death with constant suicidal thoughts. Disgusted of life and thoughts. Profound despondency. Peevish. Rapid and constant questioning without waiting for answers. Oversensitive to noise. Symptoms often worsen at night or during the winter months, but these individuals may find relief from soothing music.

Kali Phos 30C – Depressed after prolonged periods of emotional stress or excitement. It mostly helps people who are over-stressed and have much to worry about. They remain constantly sad, and gloomy. With this, they have negative thoughts in their minds. Those who need it feel mentally and physically exhausted. Mental and physical depression caused by excitement, overwork, worry and insomnia. For a person who feels depression after working too hard, being physically ill, or going through prolonged emotional stress or excitement this remedy can be helpful. Other symptoms that they may present include anxiety attacks, and spells of weeping. Exhausted, nervous and jumpy, they may have difficulty working or concentrating and become discouraged and lose confidence. Headaches from mental effort, sleeplessness, anaemia, sensitivity to the cold, and indigestion.

Sepia 30C - Is an excellent medicine to deal with cases of depression in women during menopause. The most important symptoms present in them are sadness, aversion to seeing family members, and loss of interest in doing any work either mental or physical, even missing out on daily routine activities. They also want to be alone and they may become angry when disturbed. They may feel better after crying but they prefer not to be consoled. There is also indifferent behaviour towards life and family. Such people are constantly lost in worries and are stressed with self-pity. They are very irritable and get offended easily. Sporadic weeping spells seeking consolation, and sympathy. Loss of sexual desire is another major complaint. Other related symptoms include digestion problems and menstrual issues.

Cimicifuga Racemosa 30C - Considered in cases of depression among women that begin after childbirth. Women who need this medicine suffer extreme sadness. They feel that they are enveloped in darkness from which it is difficult to come out. They also feel exhausted by these symptoms. Can be energetic and talkative when feeling well but upset and gloomy when depressed. Other symptoms can be painful menstrual periods and headaches that involve the neck, excessive talking, indifferent behaviour, fear of death, and fear of going mentally insane.

Lachesis 30C – Indicated in cases where delusion is present along with depression such as in cases of psychotic depression. Where people have sadness, feelings of being abandoned, excessive talkativeness, and delusions. Depression can be caused by jealously, suspicion, or repressed feelings, for people who dislike commitment or confinement. Indulges in excessive talking and frequently jumps from one subject to another. A lot of ideas crowd their mind at a given time. When it comes to delusions a person may get suspicious and may feel as if someone may poison or harm them. Other symptoms that appear in them are restlessness, aversion to work, and running away from the world. **A** person who worries' a lot, very talkative and experiences menopausal depression.

Arsenic Alb 30C – One of the top remedies for depression. Arsenic patients express sadness, restlessness and fear. Anxious, insecure, perfectionistic people who need this remedy may set high standards for themselves and others and become depressed if their expectations are not met. Arsenic Administered in cases where anxiety accompanies sadness. There is anxiety about health and about the future. This is attended with intense restlessness. Good remedy for excessive worriers, particularly for those that obsess about health, can be classified as a perfectionist. They often are depressed when they fail to reach personal high standards. Depression on account of a hidden feeling or guilt. Worry about material security sometimes borders on despair. Marked weakness is another prominent symptom of these. Some fears are also there like fear of disease, financial loss, being alone and of death. The person's symptoms are usually worse in colder weather, and they are also very sensitive to any pain.

Chronic Fatigue Syndrome

Chronic Fatigue Syndrome – The Centre for Disease Control and Prevention criteria for chronic fatigue syndrome is a severe fatigue lasting longer than six months, as well as presence of at least four of the following physical symptoms - post exertional malaise, unrefreshing sleep, impaired memory or concentration, muscle pain, polyarthralgia, sore throat, tender lymph nodes, or new headaches. Other symptoms can be a Low grade fever of above 100.4 °F (38°C) and chills, comes on suddenly especially after the flu, sore throat and swollen lymph glands in the neck or armpits, more common in people over age of 40, twice as many women than men are diagnosed with CFS, muscle and joint aches without any swelling, headaches, mood changes, always feels tired, sleep doesn't help, feeling as if you are in a fog and not being able to concentrate or remember and finally the condition can last a month or years. With Doctors in this disease you can wind up on anything from anti-depressants to stimulants but one good thing you can do for yourself in this time period is to sort out your diet and get it where it should be. **Nutrition** – Iridology is very useful for trying to sort out this condition and can give you plenty of clues. Some of the main clues I have seen are dark murky clouds in the eyes which suggest a toxic waste dump. These people sometimes have bowel problems and the waste is not getting out so it overloads the other systems such as the liver in trying to get rid of the waste. Some eyes have about 3 or more nerve rings so these people are under constant stress and are rapidly burning calcium and magnesium which is what the nerves live on as well as the B vitamins which are water soluble so they don't stay in the body for long. The last clue from the eye can be what is known as a Lymphatic Rosemary which means the lymph system is not removing waste from the body effectively. Nutrition wise it would be a good idea to use this time to change your diet to what it should be. Avoid refined foods, sugar, caffeine, alcohol, and saturated fats so the body can have a bit of a rest and change to more fresh vegetables, legumes, whole grains, protein, and essential fatty acids found in nuts, seeds, and cold-water fish. See the diet part of the book and go on the acid alkaline diet or even just use the superfoods mentioned there. Omega-3 fatty acids found in fish oil may also help reduce fatigue. Studies show that people with CFS have lower ratios of omega-3 to omega-6 fatty acids. Zinc for the immune system and vitamin C. For a yes or no answer when times get really bad wack the vitamin C up to about 2000 mg a day and see what happens. Vitamin C is good at getting rid of toxins and rubbish. **Herbal Treatment** – I usually start with Astragalus and Echinacea. Echinacea I would run for 3 months which is the blood cycle and then stop and reconsider the whole case again. People with Fibromyalgia should be weary in case this disease is an autoimmune one with the body attacking itself as Echinacea could build up an army just to attack itself. For males consider a very low dose like Siberian ginseng which would work more like a tonic. Panax Ginseng basically gives a shot of adrenaline to the blood which could be a bit to brutal. For females consider Withania which is another adaptogen but more female specific but good for anyone. Lemon Balm can also help in this condition and is also an Antiviral more specific to the nervous system and also used in Glandular Fever. Consider Cats Claw if you think there is an Auto immune type of problem floating around in the background.

Astragalus

Astragalus membranaceus

Actions - Immuno-modulator, anti-viral, adaptogen, hypotensive, immune stimulant, adrenal tonic, diuretic, vasodilator, cardiotonic, antioxidant, hepatoprotective, hypoglycemic.

This herb should only be used in chronic diseases, as a preventative or in cases of fatigue especially in chronic diseases. Stimulates the natural production of interferon and intensifies the white cell destruction of germs. A good tonic for strengthening the resistance to disease. Is very useful for chronic debility and fatigue by restoring the immune function. Use as a lung tonic to help expel toxins and pus in flu's, colds and sinusitis. Increases stamina and can accelerate wound healing, can help to replenish bone marrow. Strengthens the digestive system and aids adrenal gland function. This herb is used for cancer especially if the patient has had chemotherapy and helps aid them in their recovery. Thought to control body fluids such as excessive sweating, night sweats, and relieve fluid retention. Astragalus has powerful anti-aging properties slowing the aging process at a cellular level. Astragaloside IV a saponin has shown benefits in reversing cell damage and in activating telomerase, this addresses telomere shortening and slows down cellular aging. This is very important, I will try to explain. Inside every cell of your body is a Telomere, a good way to think about it is as an hour glass. Every time a cell divides it breaks a little piece of the telomere off which is a bit of sand flowing through the hour glass, when the last piece of the telomere is gone that is the last time the cell can divide, this is how we age. Now I will explain why Antioxidants are so important. Imagine a nasty little free radical with a baseball bat which has just smashed into one of your cells and is wandering round inside your cell and then comes across the telomere and says I will fix you and smashes the telomere right at the bottom and leaves only a little stump left. That's it for the cell, the life has been cut short. Astragalus root is most effective when taken long term, providing many benefits that can contribute to a longer, healthier life. Good to use for chronic fatigue syndrome (CFS) and fibromyalgia. Has cardioprotective effects helping to prevent plaque buildup in the arteries and narrowing of the blood vessel walls by protecting the inner wall of the vessel. It has also been shown to reduce blood pressure and lower triglycerides. **Immune Boosting** - Is an immunostimulant that it is known to increase the count of white blood cells and stimulate the production of antibodies, this builds up bodily resistance to viruses and bacteria. Many clinical studies have shown it boosts the immune system and encourages an increase in immune T-cells, natural killer cells, macrophages and immunoglobulin activity, production, and function. Astragalus appears to trigger immune cells from a resting state into heightened activity. The natural killer cells of the immune system also seem to be markedly enhanced to fight intruders five to six times higher than normal. **Cautions** - Should not be used in acute infections or fevers. Use with care for those with very low blood pressure. Women who are pregnant or breastfeeding should not use Astragalus. May counteract anti-diabetic agents, and potentiate effects of diuretics. People with autoimmune diseases should consult their healthcare professional before using Astragalus because of its ability to stimulate the immune system. **Part used** – Root. **Dose** - 500 to a 1000mg per day or up to 20 drops of tincture twice daily.

Homoeopathic Remedies for Chronic Fatigue Syndrome

Arsenic Album 30C - Patient feels like lying down all the time due to excessive fatigue. Standing, walking and the slightest exertion result in fatigue and lying down provides some relief to the person. Even a little exertion leads to lack of strength and weakness. Such persons also hesitate and have fear exerting because they anticipate exhaustion as a result. Apart from disabling fatigue, anxiety may also show its presence in extreme levels.

Gelsemium 30C - Indicated by weakness with drowsiness, dizziness, dullness and trembling. For mental exhaustion and indifference, physical weakness such as heaviness of the limbs and eyelids. Muscle aches with heaviness and weakness. Tremors and twitching of the muscles may also be a feature. The sufferer might have a dull heaviness in the head and have blurred vision, feels worse in damp, cold weather and mentally be dull with a lot of anxiety. Sleepiness throughout the day with disabling fatigue. Along with drowsiness and fatigue, heaviness in head may also be felt. The muscle pain is mostly present in neck, shoulders, back, hips and legs. The patient may also experience trembling and weakness in limbs.

Kali Phos 30C - A widely used remedy for CFS, especially if the illness follows influenza. The slightest mental or physical exertion leads to extreme fatigue. For such persons, even a little work seems to be a very huge task. Anxiety with depression, insomnia and nightmares. The anxiety may present as a fear of crowds and agoraphobia. Extreme prostration, weakness and tired feeling ensue from a little exertion. The person feels worn out as if all the energy has been drained out. Loss of memory might be a problem. Forgetfulness is noticeable while speaking or writing. There is muscle weakness and aches and pains, all worse with exercise, the cold and mental effort. The symptoms are better from sleep, eating and gentle movement.

You now have the information for treating Fibromyalgia – Depression and Anxiety and Fibromyalgia – Chronic Fatigue. The choice is yours to pick and choose the herbs that you think will benefit you. Every 3 months which is the blood cycle stand back and review the disease again and try to figure what worked and what hasn't, but most importantly of all is do you feel better, even a little bit. The diet for this disease is in the diet section. Now we will move along so as to help with other symptoms.

Sleep and for those with IBS

Herbs for Sleep – Chamomile is a good one to take in tea form about an hour before sleep as it will relax the body followed by Valerian in a pill form just before you sleep. Some formulas add Hops (see below) to the ones just mentioned. Ziziphus is a Chinese herb that works well and is now popular in the west.

IBS Problems - Specific herbs for IBS are Ginger and Peppermint. You can buy ginger in crystalized form which is very yummy, from mild to very hot. You can also use ginger powder to make tea and to and to improve its taste, add some lemon and little honey (Cardamom is also of the ginger family and is useful here). One of the advantages of using teas in IBS is that you have a large volume of liquid medicating a large volume of the Large intestines as it passes through. Next is Peppermint which has a proven record in treating IBS especially in the oil form (Not Essential Oil To Strong!) but the problem here is that it doesn't last so use it for only 2 weeks at a time then give it a break for the same amount of time. You can buy Peppermint oil in enteric capsules under the name of Mintec. A good herb for when the large bowel feels raw painful and maybe a bit bloated is Slippery Elm which is demulcent and soothing and coats the wall of bowel. To this add a little bit of Psyllium but not to much as it is a bulking agent used in lots of laxatives. The large bowel is big and muscular because its job is to crush all the food going through so as to recycle all the liquid so the Psyllium mixed with Slippery Elm and a bit of honey if you like will keep it busy but at the same time add a soothing protective coating to it. Also think of adding a bit of Liquorice as this also puts a soothing coating on but its coating is anti-inflammatory. Aloe Vera is another coater and soother, go to a health shop and you can buy it in one litre bottles and see if that helps and get your yes or no answer but ask them which is the best for IBS for there seems to be a lot of them around now. Another herb which you may have noticed in your research is Artichoke sold in probably powdered capsules. It has actually shown some good and interesting results and would be worth a try. Another herb to think of especially if you are having trouble sleeping is Hops which is below.

Hops

Humulus lupulus

Actions - Sedative, hypnotic, bitter, antiseptic, visceral antispasmodic, astringent, nervine.

Famed for its tonic and nervine properties, pain reliever, sleep inducer, antiseptic, tension that leads to restlessness, headache, indigestion, mucous colitis. Good for when digestive problems are caused by worry or nerves. One of the main remedies for IBS. Acts on the central nervous system and calms and eases anxiety. **Digestive System** – Nervous digestive conditions with insufficient secretions and over excitability of the nervous system. Visceral smooth muscle tensions affecting digestive and bowel functions, mucous colitis, spastic constipation, nervous dyspepsia, mucous colitis with Chamomile. Reduced stomach acidity, check fermentation. **Nervous System** – Sedative to encourage restful sleep, insomnia due to worry or nervous debility with Valerian, reduces symptoms of nervous tension, nerve pains, excitability and hysteria with Valerian. **Doses** - Tincture 1 to 4mls 3 times daily, 1 teaspoon of dried flowers in tea 3 times a day or just before bed. **Caution** - Do not use in depression.

Carpal Tunnel Syndrome

Carpal tunnel syndrome is a common condition that causes numbness, tingling, and pain in the hand and forearm. The Carpal Tunnel is in the palm side of the hand and is where the ligaments and nerves enter the hand to control the fingers. The condition begins when one of the major nerves to the hand such as the median nerve is squeezed or crushed going into the wrist from an injury. The injury can cause pain and numbness in the index and middle fingers and weakness of the thumb. Causes can be from repetitive high impact injuries to the hand from sport or occupation, crush injuries, inflammation from arthritis or rheumatism and RSI injuries especially from tools and computer keyboards. Women seem to develop this condition more than men and the condition is more common between the years 30 to 60. The disease can be associated with conditions, such as diabetes, hypothyroidism, rubella, pregnancy, connective tissues diseases, obesity, and menopause. High caffeine, tobacco, or alcohol intake may be contributing risk factors. **Symptoms** – There can be weakness when trying to grip something, pain, tingling and numbness in the areas of the fingers, hand and sometimes reaching up into the elbow, there can be pain shooting from the hand up the arm as far as the shoulder. Night time symptoms can be worse than the day pain and tingling can ruin sleep; fingers can feel useless and sometimes swollen even though there is no swelling. There can also be loss of strength in the muscle at the base of the thumb near the palm. Pain is generally caused by the compression of the median nerve though this does not explain why it is associated with all the other conditions. Some people may display clumsiness in handling objects and have a tendency to drop things. **Treatment** – Some people are given pain killers maybe along with a wrist brace and sent to physical therapy. Others with the disease more advanced may have surgery called a release which separates the ligaments in the carpal tunnel and takes the pressure off the nerve.

Nutrition – **B6** in some has improved the condition and has had a lot of research. Some studies suggest that low levels of riboflavin in the blood are associated with carpal tunnel syndrome and other inflammatory diseases. The B vitamins are water soluble and leave the body fast so maybe consider using B6 at night while you sleep as that way it's trapped in the body until you get up and pass water. For the day think of a high strength multi vitamin with slow release Bs. You will know when it's a slow release as every time you pass water the urine will look very fluorescent in colour. Eat antioxidant-rich foods, including fruits such as blueberries, cherries, tomatoes and vegetables. See the Superfoods in the diet section. Also think of the Omega-3 fatty acids such as fish oil so as to help reduce inflammation, sometimes with these I start with 2 capsules 3 times a day for 4 to 5 days especially if you have dry skin and then back it off to 3 capsules spread through the day. You should get a good yes or no if these are helping. Vitamin C at 500 to 1000 mg daily as an antioxidant can help especially if there is swelling.

Some people use Methylsulfonylmethane (MSM) 3000 mg twice a day to help reduce inflammation but I am going to use this in a different way next in the herbal treatment. **Herbal Treatment** – With conditions like this you must nip them in the bud immediately before they become a repetitive strain injury and make your life a misery. If they do, just change your occupation as it is not really worth a life time of suffering. As this condition crushes the nerves it must also do the same to the blood supply, so let's get on top of the condition at the very beginning and ruin its game plan. Here we are going to use Hot and Cold Treatment along with a formula we want to push into the affected area. The formula that we are going to use is called Glucosamine, Chondroitin and MSM in the powdered form which you should be able to find all together. The formula is very anti-inflammatory, pain relieving and also helps to build up cartilage especially after it has been worn down or out. Take the powder dissolved in about half a glass of water then wait about 15 minutes which is about when it should be entering the blood stream and then start the hot and cold water treatment. Get two buckets; fill one with hot water, as hot as you can bear and the other with very cold water. Put your wrist into the hot water for as long as you can bear, then into the cold for as long as you can bear and keep on repeating. This makes a mechanical pump, hot expands, cold contracts. You can repeat this as many times you like as you are pumping the inflammatory swelling out and freshly medicated blood in leading to decongestion and fast healing. A lot of athletes use this system and race horses don't really get much of a say in the matter, but doing this frequently during the day along with the hot and cold treatment can force heal their injuries so they can compete again as soon as possible. Our main herb here is Hypericum also known as St John's Wort which is well known for its relief given to shooting pains down nerve pathways and for its use in extreme pain conditions such as Shingles and nasty wounds in nerve rich areas. It's also an anti-depressant so you can see why they named it after a saint as it does two jobs at once. Chamomile is the next main herb as it is a nerve relaxant and loaded with Calcium and Magnesium which is what every screaming nerve needs so also consider a Calcium and Magnesium supplement. Not many people know that it is also a good anti-inflammatory. Three to four cups a day would help or you could add it to a tincture or capsule formula. Another herb to think of especially if this has turned into a Chronic Condition is Cats Claw which is used for chronic inflammatory conditions and especially if an auto immune response is suspected or the person has an underlying auto immune condition as there are still a lot of unknowns in Carpal Tunnel Syndrome. Externally Hypericum Cream can be rubbed into the affected area medicating internally and externally at the same time. An Essential Oil formula mixed into a carrier oil of Wintergreen, Chamomile and Lavender can also be used in a diluted form to help get relief. Write ups of our main herbs follow.

St John's Wort

Hypericum

Medicinal Actions - Anti-inflammatory, astringent, anti-viral, anti-spasmodic, nervine, vulnerary, antibacterial and antidepressant. St John's Wort is perhaps the most studied herb for depression with literally thousands of studies and clinical trials performed to assess its usefulness as an antidepressant. Many studies have found the herb to be equally as effective as traditional antidepressants but with fewer side effects in mild to moderately depressed patients. This is not meant to be used in major suicidal depression. Taken internally it has a sedative and pain reducing effect, which gives it a place in the treatment of neuralgia, anxiety, tension and general depression. Hyperforin which is a component of Hypericum can inhibit synaptosomal reuptake of serotonin, norepinephrine, and dopamine. It may take 2 to 4 weeks to notice clinical results when taken for depression. Useful in mild to moderate depression, anxiety, neuralgia and myalgia's and generally for pains shooting down nerve pathways. This herb is antiviral both internally and topically. **Contraindications** - Speeds up the elimination of many and can interfere with MAOIs, SSRIs, narcotics and reserpine. Do not use St. John's Wort during pregnancy or lactation. **Caution** - Photosensitivity can occur in susceptible individuals. Fair-skinned individuals should take precautions when exposed to the sun and the elderly should use protective eyewear when exposed also. **Part Used** – Aerial and flowering parts. **Dosage** – Tincture 2 to 4mls three times daily. Infusion – 1 to 2 teaspoonsful of herb infused into a cup of boiling water taken 3 times daily.

Cats Claw

Uncaria tomentosa

Actions - Anti oxidant, immune stimulant, anti-inflammatory, anti-fungal, anti-rheumatic, anti-viral, anti-tumor, hypotensive, anti-microbial.

Primary traditional uses in Peru are as an anti-inflammatory, contraceptive and anti-cancer remedy. An immune stimulant especially used in viral infections, including HIV. Useful in a variety of inflammatory diseases including gastric ulcers, diarrhea and GI tumors, gonorrhea, arthritis and rheumatism, acne, diabetes, diseases of the urinary tract and cancer. Also used to alleviate allergic sinus type conditions, boost the immune system, asthma, bursitis, Candida, immune deficiency disorders, chronic inflammatory diseases with auto immune conditions. With a lengthy history dating back to the Inca civilization, Cat's Claw has been used as a traditional medicine in the Andes to treat inflammation, gastric ulcers, rheumatism, dysentery, intestinal complaints and wounds. **Immune System** - A recent study showed that Cat's Claw significantly elevated the infection fighting white blood cell count in adult men who supplemented with this herb for 6 months. Researchers also noted a repair in DNA – both single and double strand breaks. Its effect on the immune system appears to be two fold, with the ability to both boost and dampen immune response, depending on what is needed. Hyper immune responses can be contained, whilst a weak immune system that allows disease to advance undeterred is strengthened by supplementation with Cat's Claw. **Arthritis Relief -** Multiple studies have found that Cat's Claw can be used to naturally improve osteoarthritis and rheumatoid arthritis symptoms. In a 2001 study they found that pain associated with activity, medical and pain assessment scores were significantly reduced within the first week of therapy. Another study noted that treatment with Cat's Claw extract resulted in a reduction in the number of painful joints compared with the placebo after 24 weeks of treatment. This arthritis fighting effect is thought to be from compounds that seem to be immune system modulators. **Constituents** - Cats Claw has many phytochemical elements that consist of oxidole alkaloids, quinovic acid glycosides, antioxidants, plant sterols and carboxyl alkyl esters. All of these are thought to have, in varying degrees, an action that can be attributed to the many benefits of Cats Claw. **Dose** - As labeled by supplier. **Parts used** - Inner bark of roots and stems. The bark is considered to be the most medicinally useful. Both Leaves and roots have been proven to hold significant phytochemical content but not in such concentration as is found in the bark. Traditionally the bark of Cats Claw is made into a tea or powder to be consumed over a given period depending on illness. **Contraindications** -Pregnancy, lactation or in children less than three years old **Interactions** - Typically not recommended for those taking insulin, thymus extracts, vaccines, immune globulin or sera. **Precautions** - Do not take Cat's Claw if on blood thinning medication. Large quantities can cause stomach upset because of the large number of tannins in the bark. It is recommended to increase dose in increments to lessen the symptoms of detoxification. It is not recommended to take Cat's Claw if you have scheduled surgery.

Chamomile

Matricaria recutita

Actions - Antispasmodic, nervine, sedative, carminative, anti-inflammatory, analgesic, antiseptic, allergies.

An excellent gentle sedative with a relaxing action that is good for easing anxiety and helping with sleep. Helps to restore the nervous system. It is safe to use in children and is a powerful anti-inflammatory in almost any condition and a good all round tonic for the nervous system. This is the herb for those that can worry themselves sick. As a relaxant, chamomile depresses the central nervous system, reducing anxiety while not disrupting normal performance or function. Chamomile has been used for centuries to lower pain and reduce inflammation. This seems to be backed up by science with a 2009 study finding that chamomile caused cell reactions similar to that of nonsteroidal anti-inflammatory drugs. In the digestive system it can be used for indigestion especially when there are colicky pains and is ideal for colitis and IBS type problems. For females Chamomile is good for amenorrhea, spasmodic dysmenorrhea, premenstrual irritability and menopausal tensions. This herb is also a good source of calcium and magnesium which are the nervous systems favorite minerals. **Uses** - Anxiety, colic, diverticula's, flatulence, gastritis, indigestion, insomnia, irritable, nervousness, cramps, restlessness, stress, ulcers. **Doses -** Tincture 2 to 4mls 3 times daily, for teas just the one teabag.

Homeopathic Treatment for Carpal Tunnel Syndrome

Arnica 6C to 30C - For Carpal Tunnel Syndrome that results from a wrist sprain with a bruised feeling in the wrist indicates Arnica. Sore pain when touched, wrist pain due to jar also indicates Arnica. For a bruised, beat up feeling, soreness, achy muscles after trauma or overuse. The cream form can used topically as well and can be found in most health shops.

Viola Odorata 6C to 30C – This Homeopathic Remedy is the most specific for the treatment of Carpal Tunnel Syndrome when the right wrist is affected. There is typically a pressing pain felt in the wrist, which can extend to the hand and fingers and there may be trembling in the affected hand. Pain in the right wrist after exposure to cold air and cloudy weather.

Rhus Tox 6C to 30C – Typically associated with Carpal Tunnel Syndrome from an overuse injury. Painful on beginning of movement and improves with continued movement. There is stiffness with a desire to move and stretch the wrist and hand. Pain in the right wrist increases from rest and just beginning to move is the most guiding symptoms. Cold and damp conditions aggravate the symptoms (also in Ruta cases). Carpal Tunnel Syndrome as a result of cold wet weather, before the storm, and exertion. Rheumatism with painful stiffness.

Ruta 6C to 30C – This remedy is useful in cases where strain from overuse is a factor or where a fracture or other injury is involved. Ruta has a strong affinity for tendons and ligaments. There is a sprained feeling with stiffness of the wrist and numbness and tingling after any exertion. Warmth will ease the symptoms (also in Rhus tox cases).

Calcarea Carb 6C to 30C - For Carpal Tunnel Syndrome due to wrist sprain or due to overexertion of the wrist particularly indicates Calcarea Carb. Other symptoms can be cold, clammy hands and feet.

Calc Phos 6C to 30C – The wrist feels weak and lame. This remedy is very useful in carpal tunnel syndrome if it is characterised by soreness and aching in the wrist and is aggravated by cold damp weather especially icy, snowy conditions.

Kali Carb 6C to 30C – Frequently indicated in Carpal Tunnel Syndrome, typically there are burning pains in the fingers and stitching and tearing pains in the joints and tendons. The affected arm may jerk when touched. There is numbness in the hands and forearms which is aggravated by exertion and by cold weather

Causticum 6C to 30C – One of the most frequently indicated remedies for chronic and recurring Carpal Tunnel Syndrome. There is stiffness and cramping, with burning or tearing pains in the wrist and hand. Contraction of the flexor tendons in the palm of the hand is also a typical feature. The condition is somewhat eased by warmth and warm applications. There is weakness and loss of strength in the hands, and numbness in the hands and fingers.

Bursitis

One of the main problems with this condition is that the first time it happens you usually cannot tell the difference between the pain of bursitis and the pain caused by a strain or muscle injury and would have to get medical help to sort it out. Bursae are small, jelly-like sacs that are located throughout the body in places such as the elbow, hip, knee and heel. The shoulder has a few in different places positioned between bones and soft tissues acting as cushions to help reduce friction and in the complex area of the shoulder blade it also helps the different muscles to move around each other. In the shoulder the subacromial bursae cushion is in the area between the rotator cuff tendons and the highest point of the shoulder blade. Bursae allow the tendons and bones to glide without friction when you move and lift your arms. Most of the nastiest conditions of Bursitis that I have dealt with are in the shoulder and shoulder blades with the worst being in fork lift drivers in their right shoulders as their right hand is used all the time to manipulate their levers. It is also common in truck drivers from the steering wheel and the use of forklifts. Repetitive Strain Injuries (RSI) for these workers is fairly common and is a good example of worst case conditions. In general bursitis is inflammation of the bursa. Bursitis occurs when the small fluid filled sac that helps to lubricate and cushion the joint becomes inflamed and can hurt to move. The condition usually occurs in larger joints such as the shoulder, hip, knee, or elbow and is often caused by repetitive motion. For most people bursitis usually goes away in a few weeks with treatment depending on its severity, and if it was occupationally caused. **Symptoms** – There may be redness, heat, tenderness or swelling in the affected area along with aching or stiffness in the joint, that gets worse when you move it or the pain may slowly develop gradually over time. Usually the bursa becomes irritated or injured after overuse from repetitive motion or strenuous activity. Sometimes bacterial infection may also cause bursitis along with other health problems such as gout or rheumatoid arthritis.

Treatment – Depending on where the condition is, resting and elevating the joint can sometimes help or maybe a splint, sling or support bandage or brace. A cold pack may also help to relieve the pain and swelling but the reality is you will not really know what's really happening until after a medical check-up so follow first aid procedures till then. **Herbal Treatment** – You could start with Hot and Cold Treatment using the joint formula Glucosamine, Chondroitin and MSM as mentioned in the condition above in Carpal Tunnel Syndrome but it could be a bit difficult to get your shoulder blade into a bucket of water but for the parts you can you should try it, for it is a really good and fast way for reducing inflammation. Even if you don't use the hot and cold method the Joint Formula is a good background anti-inflammatory remedy. As Bursa are basically fluid filled sacks reasonably close to the surface of the skin it is easier and faster to medicate them through the skin by using Essential Oils diluted into a carrier oil with **Boswellia** known to you as **Frankincense** being our main oil in the formula. Other oils that you can consider adding are Thyme, Eucalyptus with Ginger adding heat and to push the formula into the body.

Boswellia

Frankincense

Actions – Anti-inflammatory, anti-arthritic, analgesic, anti-rheumatic, liver protective.

A traditional remedy for wound healing and inflammatory diseases that has been used in many cultures. Also used for respiratory diseases especially the chronic ones and rheumatic disorders, diarrhoea, dysentery, piles, dysmenorrhoea and in weakness to improve the appetite and liver disorders. Studies have shown that the essential oil provides immune stimulant activity throughout the body with one study finding that Frankincense increases white blood cell production whilst keeping inflammation at a minimum. When applied topically, the oil will work to create a layer of protection against bacterial and viral infections. When inhaled the same benefits manifest internally working to heal the body from the inside out. In arthritis and rheumatism its powerful anti-inflammatory compounds such as terpenes and boswellic acids reduce joint inflammation by preventing the release of leukotrienes that can cause inflammation, with studies confirming it may be as effective as NSAIDS with no negative side effects. Frankincense essential oil can be massaged into painful joints and muscles, and has been found useful in preventing the breakdown of cartilage tissue, thus reducing inflammation. **Frankincense Essential Oil** - Frankincense essential oil is able to rejuvenate and revive tired skin and as such it is added to many beautifying lotions. Frankincense essential oil can be used in the bath, or vaporized in an oil burner. It can be added to a massage oil or cream. Use 6 to 8 drops per bath and 10 to 18 drops per 30ml of carrier oil. **Constituents -** The major constituents of Frankincense are acid resins, gum, 3-acetyl-beta-boswellic acid, alpha-boswellic acid, methyl-glucuronic acid, incensole acetate, terpines, phellandrene and pentacyclic triterpenoids. **Precautions -** None known. **Dose –** Tincture - 1 to 3 ml three times a day. Capsules 300 to 400 mg three times a day or as labelled.

Homoeopathics don't like essential oils but using Fish Oil capsules for their anti-inflammatory action especially if you have very dry skin will help. You can also keep using the Joint Formula as it will act as a good anti-inflammatory along with the fish Oil. If the **Bursitis** is caused by an infection we will add the herb Echinacea so as to boost the immune system and start taking Garlic Oil capsules which will give us a strong anti-viral and anti-bacterial response and also think of Vitamin C, maybe in 500mg and run through a bottle of that.

Echinacea
Echinacea angustifolia
Actions - Immune stimulant, anti-microbial, anti-inflammatory, alterative, healing.
This herb is an infection fighter active against strep bacteria (abscesses and boils), a blood cleanser, (blood poisons, snake bites,

poisonous insects) and a glandular and lymphatic system cleanser. Use it particularly for respiratory infections and for any disease above the waist. This is one of our main immune boosters for the acute diseases. Echinacea stimulates the bone marrow to make more white blood cells which are our main infection killers and why we only use it in short bursts. Use as a prophylactic to protect from infections especially when traveling or before going into Hospital. **Uses** - All infections, depressed immune function, inflammatory conditions, allergies, effective against both bacteria and viruses. **Dose** – 1 to 4mls of tincture. **Warning** - Do not use continually as you will burn out the immune system, give a few weeks break after 3 weeks. Beware also in the use of allergies for you could be building up the immune system just to attack itself.

Homoeopathic Treatment for Bursitis

Arnica 6C to 30C - Useful when bursitis is related to traumatic injury or strain. The affected area feels bruised and sore, and the person tries to avoid being touched, because of pain.

Belladonna 6C to 30C - Bursitis with heat and throbbing, intense discomfort caused by jarring and touch. The area often is red and swollen, and the overlying skin feels hot.

Bryonia 6C to 30C - When bursitis pain has a stitching or tearing quality and is worse from even the slightest motion, this remedy is a likely choice. The affected area is hot and swollen, feeling worse from warmth.

Ruta graveolens 6C to 30C - If bursitis is acute with swelling, great stiffness, and aching pain. Aggravated by stretching, and the person often feels fatigued or weak. Cold and dampness make it worse, lying down to rest may help.

Sanguinaria 6C to 30C - For bursitis in the shoulder especially the right shoulder. Raising the arm is difficult. Pain extends down the arm if the shoulder is moved. Worse at night in bed from lying on the affected part, and also when turning over.

Sprains Strains and Tendonitis

Here we will deal with Sprains, Strains and Tendonitis will follow mainly so that we can clearly see the differences in the symptoms, conditions and severity. Sprains and strains are usually minor injuries that often occur during sports, exercise, or other physical activity. A sprain is an injury to a ligament which is the tissue that links bones together at the joints. Sprains happen most often in the ankle, knee, elbow, or wrist. The difference between a sprain and a strain is that a sprain injures the bands of tissue that connect two bones together, while a strain is an injury to a muscle, or to the band of tissue that attaches a muscle to the bone. Strains are tears in muscle tissue. They happen most often in the muscles that support the calf, thigh, groin, and shoulder. Sometimes sprains and strains can be severe, and require weeks of rehabilitation. Tendinitis is an **inflammation of the thick fibrous cords that attach muscle to bone**. These cords are called tendons. The main symptom is pain and tenderness right outside a joint and around it. Often happens as a result of repetitive movements and can become chronic if ignored and not treated. Common areas for tendinitis are often the shoulder which is known as rotator cuff tendinitis, with others being tennis elbow or golfer's elbow along with wrist injuries. Most of these conditions can easily turn into Repetitive Strain Injuries if not dealt with properly and given time to heal. Carpel Tunnel is a good example of what can happen if you don't give injuries a chance to heal properly. But never fear we have our MSM Joint formula (see write up in the diet section) and hot and cold treatment to speed the way for us in this impatient and fast moving world that does not give us the time to heal properly. **Symptoms** – Can be muscle stiffness, tenderness, soreness and swelling, with sprains there can be bruising as well. You will soon know how bad the problem is when you try to use it. Cold water, icepack or even a pack of frozen peas should be thought of immediately. If the injury is unstable after the cold treatment then an xray may be needed. Ice reduces pain, bleeding, and inflammation but do not let it come into direct contact with the skin, wrap a cloth or folded tea towel over the area first.

If you have severe tendinitis that is not healing you may need surgery. **Treatment** – For the more severe injuries after the cold treatment we use our main Joint formula **Glucosamine Sulphate, Chondroitin Sulphate and (MSM) Formula** along with what is known as Hot and Cold Treatment especially for ankles. Wait for about 20 minutes so as to allow the formula to get into the blood stream. It works like this, put the swollen ankle in a bucket of hot water, as hot as they can bare and there leave for about 3 to 5 minutes then put in a bucket of very cold water for 3 to 5 minutes, keep repeating the process. This works like a mechanical pump eg hot expands then cold contracts, so you are pumping the inflammatory swelling out and fresh blood in leading to decongestion and fast healing. Glucosamine is an anti-inflammatory while the chondroitin helps rebuild cartilage and heal joints and attachments. You use this in the powdered form dissolved in water as it is rapidly absorbed by the intestine and enters the blood which takes it to the injury by means of the hot and cold pump. A lot of athletes and horses use this frequently during the day along with the hot and cold treatment to force heal their injuries so they can compete again as soon as possible. Three times a day is good enough for the rest of us. **Herbal Treatment** - For a bad sprain or strain I would use lots of Arnica cream to start with which will start dealing with the bruising and at night I would apply Arnica and Comfrey mixed creams along with a support bandage for the area so as to keep the cream there and also for the extra heat to the area that would create. If you grow Comfrey in your garden then you could put on a Comfrey poultice at night. Ginger is another herb that could be used in a poultice at night. If there is still a lot of swellings carry on using the hot and cold treatment along with the joint formula. When dealing with tendonitis, you don't usually think to turn to herbs. One such herb that helps reduce inflammation is Turmeric mainly by one of its chemicals called curcumin. Other herbs to help ease the pain of tendonitis are Boswellia, White Willow which is a pain killer and Ginger along with Devil's Claw. Ginger is an anti-inflammatory herb has pain relieving properties and works by slowing the production of the inflammatory compounds such as prostaglandin and leukotriene. It also helps to block the transmission of pain signals.

Boswellia comes from India and is traditionally used as an anti-inflammatory, its boswellic acids have an anti-inflammatory response. The herb is also known as Frankincense so it can also be used in the Essential Oils form along with Ginger.

Turmeric

Curcuma long

Actions – Anti-inflammatory, anti-oxidant, anti-cancer, anti-biotic and microbial, circulatory stimulant, alterative, liver restorative and protector.

This was kind of the forgotten herb that has now rocketed on to the market. I think most of the old Western Herbalists decided they would just use Ginger as Turmeric comes from the same family. We will start with Arthritis where it is very helpful with pain relief due to its powerful anti-inflammatory effects, so it will help with Rheumatism to. Used also in Tendonitis, Bursitis and generally for any pain accompanied by inflammation. Turmerics antibacterial properties can help to heal wounds and skin abrasions and also help in the pain of these conditions. Used for liver and digestive complaints where it increases liver function and helps with jaundice and promotes liver function and bile production along with protecting the liver from toxic agents. Turmeric is also a useful digestive aid to relieve flatulence and to protect the stomach mucosa against ulceration and also moderates insulin response. Turmeric has also been linked to improving brain function, especially in the areas of memory and attention span, curcumin is one of the main active chemicals that have been shown to boost levels of the brain hormone BDNF, which increases the growth of new neurons and fights various degenerative processes in the brain. Being a powerful antioxidant which neutralises damaging free radicals, it also increases the activity of the body's own antioxidant enzymes and stimulates the body's own antioxidant mechanisms against free radicals which is also good for heart health. Curcumin improves the function of endothelium which is the lining of the blood vessels. Endothelium dysfunction is a well-known cause for heart disease as it is what the plaques stick to and damage causing the blockages in the arteries. Curcumin interferes with intestinal cholesterol-uptake by increasing the conversion of cholesterol into bile acids by the liver which is another bonus to the heart. Turmeric can be an immune-booster and has also been shown to be cytotoxic to cancer and may be used to prevent and to treat cancer. This herb has been used in India for thousands of years, especially in foods and is one of the main ingredients in curry. As one of the main Ayurveda herbs it is used as a digestive, circulatory, and respiratory stimulant and is said to be cleansing for the chakras and purifying the body. **Constituents** - Turmeric contains Curcuminoids and a volatile oil containing turmerone, zingiberene, cineole and monoterpenes. Vitamins - Especially rich in B vitamins and C, B2, B3, B6, Folate. Minerals - Potassium, Phosphorus, Magnesium, Calcium, Iron, Zinc, Copper and Manganese. **Precautions** - Turmeric can cause heartburn, stomach cramps or nausea. Take caution if you have gallstones. May also cause skin rashes in sensitive individuals and may increase sensitivity to sunlight in large doses. **Parts used-** Rhizome. **Dosage** – I have decided not to give any as all the dosages seem to be different and it is used in so many ways especially in foods, so follow what the label says as hopefully they will know the strength they are using it in.

Homoeopathic Treatment

Joint problems due to twisting, wrenching or over use. A sprain can be damaged tendons or ligaments when the connecting tissues around a joint are over stretched. This can also damage the surrounding skin and fine capillaries and blood vessels causing bruising. Use your normal first aid procedures and support the joint with bandage and give the appropriate remedies with the first one being Arnica. If there is no sign of improvement in 24 to 36 hours get checked for a fracture or other damage.

Arnica 6C - For the shock and bruised sore pains. Arnica cream can also be applied as long as the skin is not broken.

Bellis Perennis 6C - Deeper acting then Arnica, intense soreness of the muscles, where swellings and lumps remain after the injury.

Ledum 6C - Injuries where the swollen part is cold or numb, sometimes looks purple and puffy, feels better for cold applications.

Ruta 6C - If the bones inside or near the joint feel bruised.

Anti-Inflammatory and Anti Rheumatic Herbs

These herbs are of two major types those that are anti-inflammatory by being the precursors of cortisone eg licorice, wild yam and devils claw. The others are anti-inflammatory but from their salicin content which is anodyne and reduces heat and swelling eg Meadowsweet, white and black willow bark and to a lesser extent poplar bark. Some arthritics should avoid herbs with salcins if they are sensitive to aspirins.

Cortisonal Herbs

Licorice Stimulates the immune system, demulcent, emollient, laxative, expectorant, antispasmodic, anti-inflammatory, adrenal agent, arthritic and rheumatic problems, inflammations especially of the GIT, colic, ulcers, gastritis.

Caution - May produce cortisone intolerance, - depleting K and Na retentive leading to hypertension, don't use with blood pressure pills.

Wild Yam

Spasmolytic, anti-inflammatory, anti-rheumatic contains a alkaloid similar to cocaine - diascorine which is anti-spasmodic and anodyne. Specific for sharp rheumatic pains of sharp twisting type that change position, stimulates removal of wastes especially from joints, useful for cramping especially in the legs, rheumatic and inflammatory conditions.

Devils Claw

Actions - Anti-inflammatory, anti-rheumatic, analgesic, sedative, diuretic and antioxidant, bitter, hepatic.

Specific for rheumatic and other joint diseases, arthritis, pain and muscle pain, lumbago, tendonitis, gout, inflammation of connective tissues. Has significant anti-inflammatory activity. Can be used in tendonitis and to treat degenerative diseases of the musculoskeletal system. Affects, liver, stomach, joints, kidneys a blood cleanser, removes deposits in joints, aids in the elimination of uric acid from the body.

Dosage - As on bottle. 1 to 2mls of tincture 3 times daily.

Salicin Based Anti-Inflammatory Herbs

Meadowsweet

See tonics, uses - inflammatory conditions, a major tonic for rheumatic conditions, muscle and joint pain, anti-rheumatic, diuretic, diaphoretic, analgesic, antiseptic in acid conditions.

White Willow Bark
Tonic, febrifuge, anti-rheumatic, anti-periodic, astringent, anti-inflammatory, analgesic, antiseptic, diuretic.
Uses - specific for rheumatoid arthritis and connective tissue disorders with inflammatory changes, gouty arthritis, neuralgias, bleeding wounds, eczema.

Analgesic Herbs

The main role of these herbs is to give pain relief while the longer acting and more therapeutic herbs begin to work on the disease itself. They are for temporary use only. The most useful ones for arthritic conditions are - St John's Wort, Jamaican Dogwood, Valerian, Rhus Tox and the Homoeopathic tincture of Apis, Salicin herbs are also analgesic.

Jamica Dogwood
Sedative, anodyne, spasmolytic, strong respiratory stimulant, anti-inflammatory, specific for insomnia due to neuralgia or nervous tension, useful for arthritic and rheumatic conditions for its anodyne and spasmolytic effects. Caution - can produce gastric distress and nausea.

Diuretic and Other Useful Anti Rheumatic Herbs

Celery Seed
Anti-rheumatic, sedative, urinary antiseptic, diuretic, tonic, diaphoretic, carminative, uterine stimulant increases uric acid elimination and possibly other acids via the kidneys.
Specific - rheumatoid arthritis with mental depression, arthritic conditions associated with acidic accumulation's, gout, dysmenorrhea, promotes restfulness and sleep, mild stimulant to system, dropsical conditions, liver problems, neuralgia, use with Menyanthes and or Guaiacum for rheumatic conditions.

Bogbean Menyanthes Trifoliata

Bitter digestive stimulant, stimulating laxative, anti-inflammatory diuretic, cholagogue, anti-rheumatic. Rheumatoid arthritis associated with digestive and disability, chronic inflammatory conditions, auto immune diseases.

Black Cohosh

Anti-spasmodic, alterative, tonic, vasodilator, diaphoretic, muscular rheumatism, neuralgias, muscle cramps, myalgia, any inflammatory condition associated with spasm or tension.

Diet and Nutrition
Muscular Skeletal System

Here we look at the diets suitable for the muscular skeletal system. The main diet I always push is the Acid and Alkaline diet, mainly because most of the people I see with cancer or severe chronic diseases, when I show them Acid and Alkaline chart they are mainly in the acid side. This makes the diet perfect for the Muscular Skeletal System as most of the serious diseases are caused by acid with good examples being Gout and Rheumatism. We will carry on using these two diseases as they are acid based diseases. When we have these diseases we have too much acid in the system with the main culprits being a diet of too much sugar, protein, alcohol and or artificial sweeteners. What makes matters worse are the body will try to use calcium and magnesium and anything it can get its hands on to buffer the acid as the blood has to be always slightly alkaline to do its work. This now creates new problems with the obvious one being for those with Osteoporosis who already have calcium deficiencies. So you need to find out if you are living in the acid lane or the alkaline.

Diet and Nutrition

For those of us getting old as you age you generate less saliva and stomach acid making it more difficult for your body to process certain vitamins and minerals, such as B12, B6 and folic acid, which are necessary to maintain mental alertness, good memory and good circulation. Your taste and smell senses diminishes with age and you lose sensitivity to salty and bitter tastes so you have to be careful not to over salt your food. To all you young ones enjoy it while you can as time tends to go by fast and then it's too late. Time to get back to the basics. First as we age we tend to put on weight because the metabolism is slowing down and food doesn't pass through the system as fast as it used to, which means the body has more time to absorb fat and everything else you don't want it to. For the younger ones you reach your peak at about 36. Next we may not be using as much energy as what we used to for example females after menopause require many hundreds of calories less than before because the body does not need the energy any more to keep the monthly cycle going, so if you are female and in menopause and eat what you have always eaten you will most likely be putting on weight. The benefits of healthy eating include increased mental acuteness, resistance to illness and disease, higher energy levels, faster recuperation times, and better management of chronic health problems, so let's get back to basics. Concentrate buying your food from Vegetable and Fruit shops or the local markets and go back to using the local butcher. Avoid processed foods as they are loaded with the wrong types of fat and too much salt and sugar. Use the supermarket for all your other needs. Just by doing this you are half way there and are keeping a lot of your money in your local community. Malnutrition is your worst enemy as it depletes your body of its reserves and lowers your immune response and the other enemy can be a lower income which is another good reason for going back to basics. Remember the old saying let your foods be your medicines and your medicines be your foods, well now is the time to put it in practice.

Calories needed for adults of different ages.

Use the following as guidelines but remember it is not taking size into account, so big people may need more and little less.

For Women

A woman over 50 who is:

Not physically active needs about 1600 calories a day.

Somewhat physically active needs about 1800 calories a day.

Very active needs about 2000 calories a day.

A woman over 30 to 50 who is:

Not physically active needs about 1800 calories a day.

Somewhat physically active needs about 2000 calories a day.

Very active needs about 2200 calories a day.

A woman over 19 to 30 who is:

Not physically active needs about 2000 calories a day.

Somewhat physically active needs about 2000 to 2200 calories a day.

Very active needs about 2400 calories a day.

For Men

A man over 50 who is:

Not physically active needs about 2000 calories a day.

Somewhat physically active needs about 2200 to 2400 calories a day.

Very active needs about 2400 to 2800 calories a day.

A man over 30 to 50 who is:

Not physically active needs about 2200 calories a day.

Somewhat physically active needs about 2400 to 2600 calories a day.

Very active needs about 2400 to 2800 calories a day.

A man over 19 to 30 who is:

Not physically active needs about 2400 calories a day.

Somewhat physically active needs about 2600 to 2800 calories a day.

Very active needs about 3000 calories a day.

Overview of your new Diet

In reality diets usually don't work. What happens is that people go on a diet then go back to what they normally do and back comes the weight, meanwhile our primitive metabolism is thinking wow that was a really bad famine back there, I better store heaps of fat for next year in case there is another famine. The only diets that work are a change in lifestyle and eating habits. As mentioned before get off the processed foods and your half way there. The easiest way to replace old habits is to replace them with new habits, this is the least traumatic way of going about it and at least you will know what the new habits are for. Next is to know yourself and your weaknesses. Regard this statement in the mental and physical. Sticking to the physical and medical point of view we want to make your new diet suited to your weak areas and medical liabilities. You may be genetically programmed and susceptible to cardiovascular disease, Rheumatism and Arthritis or Cancer could be very strong in your family or for male's Prostrate problems, so sticking to your foods being your medicines we want to base your diet on preventing and helping your medical liabilities, but we will go into more detail about that later. Your main focus for your new diet will be low carbohydrate foods, nutritious foods, foods that are high in fibre and moderately lean protein, notice I didn't say lean like all the others do, this is because the high fibre will lower the cholesterol so always remember this for it is one of the main faults of a processed food diet which generally lacks fibre. If you like cooking like me then you know fat is where the flavour is, so where there is animal fat always add fibre and this will lower the cholesterol the body can absorb. Another consideration should be the elimination of refined sugar and refined flour products. Yes I know it's hard but you could do what I do and use honey as my main sweetener its good in teas (sugar substitutes are Stevia, Sorbitol, Allulose, use in small doses)   and as for refined flour, well we all know you can make glue using flour and water, and this is what it does inside of you as well as being responsible for most of the constipation people suffer from. Try to use unrefined preferably organic wholegrain products such as whole meal bread, whole meal flour for cakes, biscuits etc, whole meal pasta, and brown rice.

Protein - Is the building blocks of the body and is required for the ongoing repair of the body. When I used to work in chemists helping people with their dieting I was taught that a general mug proof way of telling people their daily requirements of protein is that it is a palm sized piece of steak or other protein. Minus the fingers and thumb, you want it about the size of the remaining palm and the same thickness of the palm. This is a good and easy way to remember as it suits everyone because a little four foot ladies palm is in proportion to her body, and it's the same for a big seven foot male. It is best to have protein at every meal because protein is hard to digest and requires energy to do so, and when it is all chewed up in the mouth and mixed up with all the other food it forces digestion to go slowly and makes you feel fill longer. Compare this to a simple carbohydrate which is as the name suggests, simple to digest so the body only needs minutes for this and is rewarded with lot of energy. This is the mechanics of the body. Protein rich food being digested has to be digested slower because it is more complex and harder for the body to do, use this to your advantage by having protein with every meal and slow down the digestive process and sugar release, and feel full for longer. This can also save you from Diabetes. The metabolic breakdown of protein produces uric acid so for those with rheumatism, arthritis and gout bear this in mind for a lot of your treatment is aimed at reducing acid so you don't want to go much past your daily requirements. Forms of protein are red meat, poultry, fish, beans, peas, eggs, nuts, seeds, dairy and cheese.

Carbohydrates - Concentrate on the complex carbohydrates rather that the simple carbohydrates, for simple are mainly found in processed foods and release their sugar fast for energy and are part of the reason diabetes is so prevalent now. A good example is white bread. Complex carbohydrates release their sugars slowly because that is what they are complex, so the body has to spend time pulling them to pieces, lots of them are full of fibre which helps to protect us from too much cholesterol and also keeps the bowel moving so complex carbohydrates are a win situation.

Foods to Pay Attention to

Here we will start by explaining what GI is. GI is an abbreviation for Glycaemic Index which is basically the sugar value of each food determined by the rise in blood sugar. High GI is usually found in simple carbohydrates with Low GI found in complex carbohydrates. After the food will be a number which is its GI value, I will start with the high numbers and work down to the low, I am just giving you a small example; you should be able to find lots more low GI foods for your area in the correct seasons.

Low GI = 53 or less

Medium GI = 56 - 69

High GI = 70 or more

Below is just a small list of foods to give you ideas, I will leave it to you to research all the low GI foods that you like and match them to your other favourite foods. There are hundreds of books out there that give you the GI of nearly every food there is. Just go through them and choose what you like.

Vegetables - Dark green leafy vegetables are nutrient rich such as spinach and broccoli as well as the yellow and orange vegetables such as carrots, squash and yams. Try to avoid the energy rich ones or high GI ones such as potatoes or eat them in moderation with other complex carbohydrates so as to slow down their sugar release.

Low GI - Sweet corn 47, boiled carrots 41, green peas 39, raw carrots 16, eggplant 15, cauliflower 15, tomatoes 15, green beans 15, broccoli 10, cabbage 10, mushrooms 10, chilies 10, lettuce 10, red peppers 10, onions 10.

Fruits - Try not to have juices as they are generally loaded with extra sugar so focus on whole fruit for the fibre and nutrients especially the more colourful ones as they are usually the ones high in antioxidants.

Low GI - Kiwi fruit 47, coconut 45, grapes 43, pears 41, strawberries 40, oranges 40, apples 34, dried apricots 32, prunes 29, peaches 28, grapefruit 25, plums 24, cherries 22.

Grains - Always go for the whole grains as you get the fibre and they are generally complex carbohydrates so you also get the slow sugar release and stay full longer. White bread has a GI of 71 while soya and linseed bread is 36 GI

Bread Example - Sour dough wheat 54, whole wheat 49, sour dough rye 48, wholegrain pumpernickel 46, heavy mixed grain 45, soya and linseed 36.

Diet, Cancer and Chronic Diseases and Acid

I now believe one of the main causes of cancer is from the body being constantly acidic. It is said Disease and Cancer are found in Acid bodies, it is also said Cancer can't live in an alkaline body. My training as an Iridologist taught me to see what acid eyes look like and the constant contacts of people with cancer over the years slowly lead me to this conclusion. So a long time ago I made my own Acid and Alkaline Chart as it was the only way I could get one at the time.

For way over a decade everyone with cancer was shown the chart and we tried to work out where their diet was and nearly all the time they were in the acid areas of the chart or as I refer to it, in the acid lane or living in the acid lane. At that time I was in a very large Pharmacy in the middle of a state capital city for a number of years where I had dealings with literally thousands of people with lots of them being tourists. Anyone with cancer was shown the chart and had it explained to them with the result of most of them being in the acid lane, not only in food but usually from stress, worry and overwork. Anger also raises the acid levels and to make it worse, I have seen many who are angry at getting Cancer and even more angry that their body has betrayed them, and who's going to look after my young family now. They stand in front of me with their fists clenched tight and you can almost feel the rage, this is not fair, it's not right, what am I going to do, who will look after my family. Using this as an example you can see why you have to remove the cause before any real healing can begin and give them hope. You have to explain to them what their rage and diet is doing to them. Someone with that amount of anger and stress is rapidly using up all their B vitamins, along with calcium and magnesium which the nervous system would be gobbling up at a fast rate, as its taking most of the burden from the stress and then imagine how much adrenaline must be in the blood of one so angry, so that's more B vitamins being used to support that system and a massive raise in blood pressure. Let's move this case further along and see what else is happening. Human blood is always slightly alkaline, if it goes into the acid we die of what is called Acidosis. So if you are living in the acid lane and your blood is in a constant battle to keep itself in the alkaline lane, then the body is in constant stress which makes more acid, but it has no choice but to keep itself-alkaline, so to do that it has to use the minerals in the body to buffer that acid, with the main ones being Calcium and Magnesium. Can you see the vicious circle? So imagine a lifetime in the acid lane, living on processed food and fizzy drinks which are pumped full of carbonic acid to make the bubbles and loaded with sugar which breaks down to acid, and you get the sad picture of lots of people with cancer and lots of people with osteoporosis, because the blood has had to steal its Calcium and Magnesium from the bones because it's taken it from every other place as much as it can without breaking down the system. Sometimes the chemist has sent over to me people with cancer who are obviously close to the end of their time and I have shown them the chart, explained it and then given them a photocopy of it and a couple of months later they will pop up and come and see me and say they think it has helped them a bit but by this time it is usually to late the damage is done, but they do appreciate the company and having someone to talk to and I know they will be showing the chart to others and talking about it. Let's now start to get to know the chart. I am happy to say that a lot more people are of the same opinion now so you should be able to find a lot more information on the internet and a few downloadable charts.

Guide to the Chart

Excessively acid bodies try to make themselves more Alkaline so they tend to use what is easily available to do this which is usually Calcium and Magnesium which do a good job of buffering acid. Too much protein puts acid in the system, mainly uric acid which results from the breakdown of protein. White sugar put lots of acid in the body along with alcohol, which when you break it down is just sugar. Disease and Cancer are found in Acid bodies, it is said Cancer can't live in an alkaline body. Use alkaline foods to correct the imbalance. This is what the chart is for, it allows you to see if your diet is to acid and it shows you how to change it by eating more alkaline foods and reducing the acid foods.

1. - Human blood pH should be slightly alkaline (7.35 - 7.45). A pH of 7.0 is neutral. A pH below 7.0 is acidic. A pH above 7.0 is alkaline. A blood pH of 6.9, which is only slightly acidic, can induce coma and death.

2. - An acidic pH can occur from, an acid forming diet, emotional stress, toxic overload, immune reactions or any process that deprives the cells of oxygen and other nutrients. The body will try to compensate for acidic pH by using alkaline minerals. If the diet does not contain enough minerals to compensate, a build-up of acids in the cells will occur.

3. - Alkaline or Acid forming describes the ash residue after metabolism. Citrus tastes acidic but leaves an alkaline residue.

4. - Disease and Cancer are found in Acid bodies, it is said Cancer can't live in an Alkaline body. Use alkaline foods to correct the imbalance.

5. - Most people eat acid producing processed foods like white flour and sugar and drink acid producing beverages like coffee and soft drinks. We use too many drugs, which are acid forming; and we use artificial sweeteners which really wack up the acid levels.

6. - To maintain health, the diet should consist of 60% alkaline forming foods and 40% acid forming foods. To restore health, the diet should consist of 80% alkaline forming foods and 20% acid forming foods.

7. - Generally, alkaline forming foods include: most fruits, green vegetables, peas, beans, lentils, spices, herbs and seasonings, and seeds and nuts.

8. - Generally, acid forming foods include: meat, fish, poultry, eggs, grains, refined sugar and legumes.

9. - Protein foods combine well with vegetables but not starches. Starches combine well with other vegetables and also light protein such as dairy foods.

10. - Fruit is best on its own. For digestive distress use Lemon juice as this is a great alkalizer.

11. - Try to make the diet 80% alkaline and 20% acid when you start using the chart. Lemon can be added to sauces, casseroles and fish to reduce acid. Nibble on dates etc.

12. - Add lemon juice to the fridge cold water so every time you drink it you are alkalizing the body.

13. - Rest, sleep and exercise are all alkalizers while the negative emotions make acid. Remember to eat according to your occupation.

14. - Deep breathing releases at least 50% of body toxins so set a time aside each day to do this for a while. Remember happy cells don't mutate.

Herbs - Some of the best herbal digestive remedies are Ginger, Peppermint, Chamomile and Dandelion; these can be made as a tea. Apple Cider Vinegar or Lemon can be added to the teas for their alkalizing effect. Foods can be cooked with herbs for those with poor tummies. Think of the mentioned herbs and then add Fennel, Anise, Cayenne, Dill, Garlic, Parsley, Fenugreek, Curry etc. See a Herbalist for Herbs more suited to your condition.

The Acid and Alkaline Chart

For protection against and to help Cancer, Osteoporosis and Chronic Diseases use the Acid and Alkaline Chart. I will repeat this again close to the chart so you can go back and forth easily. Excessively acid bodies try to make themselves more Alkaline so they tend to use what is easily available to do this which is usually Calcium and Magnesium which do a good job of buffering acid. Too much protein puts acid in the system, mainly uric acid which results from the breakdown of protein. Sugar also put lots of acid in the body along with alcohol which also enhances inflammatory conditions. Disease and Cancer are found in Acid bodies, it is said Cancer can't live in an Alkaline body. Use alkaline foods to correct the imbalance. This is what the chart is for, it allows you to see if your diet is to acid and it shows you how to change it by eating more alkaline foods and reducing the acid foods. Diet is very important, consider this, every 3 months the blood replaces itself, every year the bones replace themselves. In a year's time are you going to have a healthy body or a junk food body? Don't forget if you eat on the acid side the bones won't be all that strong anyway.

Extremely Acid Forming Foods - pH 5.0 to 5.5

5.0 - Artificial sweeteners, Overwork, Fear, Stress, Anger, Jealously.

5.5 - Beef, Carbonated soft drinks and fizzy drinks, Cigarettes (tailor made), Drugs, Flour (white, wheat), Goat, Lamb, Pastries and cakes from white flour, Pork, Sugar (white), Beer, Brown sugar, Chicken, Deer, Chocolate, Coffee, Custard with white sugar, Jams, Jellies, Liquor, Pasta (white), Rabbit, Semolina, Table salt refined and iodized, Tea black, Turkey, Wheat bread, White rice, White vinegar (processed).

Moderate Acid - pH 6.0 to 6.5

6.0 - Cigarette tobacco (roll your own), Fish, Fruit juices with sugar, Maple syrup (processed), Pickles (commercial), Shellfish, Breads (refined) of corn, oats, rice and rye, Cereals (refined) e.g. Weetabix, corn flakes, Wheat germ, Whole Wheat foods, Wine, Yogurt (sweetened).

6.5 - Bananas (green), Buckwheat, Cheeses (sharp), Corn and rice breads, Egg whole (cooked hard), Ketchup, Mayonnaise, Oats, Pasta (whole grain), Pastry (wholegrain and honey), Peanuts, Potatoes (with no skins), Popcorn (with salt and butter), Rice (basmati), Rice (brown), Soy sauce (commercial), Tapioca, Wheat bread (sprouted organic).

Slightly Acid to Neutral pH 7.0

7.0 - Barley malt syrup, Barley, Bran, Cashews, Cereals, (unrefined with honey-fruit-maple syrup), Cornmeal, Cranberries, Fructose, Honey (pasteurized), Lentils, Macadamias, Maple syrup (unprocessed), Milk (homogenized) and most processed dairy products, Nutmeg, Mustard, Pistachios, Popcorn and butter, (plain), Rice or wheat crackers (unrefined), Rye (grain), Rye bread (organic sprouted), Seeds, (pumpkin and sunflower), Walnuts, Blueberries, Brazil nuts, Butter (salted), Cheeses, (mild and crumbly), Crackers (unrefined rye), Dried beans, Dry coconut, Egg whites, Goats milk (homogenized), Olives (pickled), Pecans, Plums, Prunes.

Slightly Alkaline to Neutral pH 7.0

7.0 – Almonds, Artichokes (Jerusalem), Barley-Malt, Brown Rice Syrup, Brussels Sprouts, Cherries, Coconut (fresh), Cucumbers, Eggplant, Honey (raw), Leeks, Miso, Mushrooms, Okra, Olives ripe, Onions, Pickles, (homemade), Radish, Sea salt, Spices, Taro, Tomatoes, (sweet), Vinegar (sweet brown rice), Water Chestnut, Artichoke (globe), Chestnuts (dry roasted), Egg yolks (soft cooked), Goat's milk and whey (raw), Horseradish, Mayonnaise (homemade), Millet, Olive oil, Rhubarb, Sesame seeds (whole), Soy beans (dry), Soy cheese, Soy milk, Sprouted grains, Tofu, Tomatoes (less sweet), Yeast, (nutritional flakes)

Moderate Alkaline - pH 7.5 to 8.0

8.0 - Apples (sweet), Apricots, Alfalfa sprouts, Arrowroot, Flour, Avocados, Bananas (ripe), Berries, Carrots, Celery, Currants, Dates and figs, (fresh), Garlic, Gooseberry, Grapes (less sweet), Grapefruit, Guavas, Herbs (leafy green), Lettuce, (leafy green), Nectarine, Peaches (sweet), Pears, (less sweet), Peas (fresh sweet), Pumpkin (sweet), Sea salt (vegetable), Spinach

7.5 - Apples (sour), Bamboo shoots, Beans (fresh green), Beets, Bell Pepper, Broccoli, Cabbage; Cauliflower, Carob, Daikon, Ginger (fresh), Grapes (sour), Kale, Lettuce (pale green), Oranges, Parsnip, Peaches (less sweet), Peas (less sweet), Potatoes and skin, Pumpkin (less sweet), Raspberry, Strawberry, Squash, Sweet corn (fresh), Tamari, Turnip, Vinegar (apple cider)

Extremely Alkaline Forming Foods - pH 8.5 to 9.0

8.5 - Agar, Cantaloupe, Cayenne (Capsicum),Dried dates and figs, Kelp, Limes, Mango, Melons, Papaya, Parsley, Seedless grapes, (sweet), Watercress, Seaweeds, Asparagus, Endive, Kiwifruit, Fruit juices, Grapes (sweet), Passion fruit, Pears (sweet), Pineapple, Raisins, Vegetable juices

9.0 – Lemons and Watermelon.

This was my main chart a long time ago and no doubt there are a few mistakes in it but over time I decided to leave the numbers alone as they can often confuse people and I currently use charts that say HIGHLY ALKALINE, MODERATELY ALKALINE, LOW ALKALINE etc and have lists of foods under each heading. One that I use often now to help people is called Alkaline Food Chart and on another page is Acidic Food Chart and I put them back to back and laminate them which give me an easy to use tool. There are lots to choose from now on the internet; I generally use about 4 of my favourites which give me more foods to choose from. As mentioned before diets don't really work mainly because you soon get back to your old habits when you finish, but this is different as you are doing this for medical reasons and all the foods are natural and healthy and you have the choice to combine them any way you want. As you are not really eating processed foods anymore buy all your fruit and veg locally and use your local butcher and baker and keep all your money in your local community.

The Diet Reality We Live In

The reality is, if you want a healthy diet avoid processed foods. I was reading an article about how the Health System could collapse in the USA because of all the chronic disease in the population and the article ended saying we haven't really got a medical crisis we have a diet crisis. If we fixed the diet there would be no medical crisis. It's amazing how such a simple and obvious truth will probably never be fixed and possibly destroys the Western Worlds Medical system. Let's start with the most obvious problem which is how many people are overweight. The World Health Organization says that 39% of adults aged 18 years and over were overweight in 2016, and 13% were obese. I think we can add at least 3 to 4 percent to that figure at the least to bring it up to modern times. Our western diet of processed foods are loaded with sugar and salt along with nitrates, artificial food colours, preservatives and lots of saturated fats. Salt alone leads to fluid retention which can make it hard to breathe for people with lung problems (only use Vegetable Salt and you will half you dose immediately). We all like fried foods such as chips loaded with fat and salt that can also cause bloating, which pushes the stomach into the diaphragm which crushes the lungs reducing air intake and if you are overweight every time you bend forward your tummy would push into the diaphragm reducing air and possibly causing gastric reflux as well. After Salt and Fat comes the Sugar and we all know what that does, but it is interesting to note that advertising caters to our cravings, which leads to mass production, which then leads to all the processed foods having to be loaded with more chemicals so as to increase their shelf life and make their colours look natural. We are our own worst enemies. One of my biggest gripes is about white bread which most of the Western World eats and lives on, is that it is nutritionally just carbohydrates for energy. Also consider bread is mostly flour and water (no fibre) which is of course our first glue, and that is exactly what it does inside the body, now known as constipation. When I was a kid I can remember an elderly Maori man telling us, white man is a fool as he grinds the wheat and uses the white flour to make bread and gives all the husks and waste to the Donkeys, now the white men are getting smaller and the donkeys are getting bigger. The reality is if we want to be healthy we first have to get to our right weight. I push the Acid Alkaline diet as it's fairly obvious when you see sick people and investigate their diets, they live mostly in the acid lane. This diet gets people back on to natural foods fast and sometimes gives them fast results.

Drink plenty of Water

This really depends on the climate you are in and what you do for work as a construction worker would need more than an office worker. About 1 and a half to 2 litres a day is a good goal but take lots more on hot days especially in summer. Some people fill a water pitcher every morning with all the water they are supposed to drink in one day and spread it out over the entire day. The human body is made up of 50 to 65 percent of water, which indicates how important it is to the body. Water helps control and regulates our body temperature, keeping it in check so that our brain and vital organs don't overheat or get too cold and maintains the balance of bodily fluids. It allows for the circulation of these fluids within the body, such as our blood, lymph and digestive fluids. Water provides a medium for the body to transport and assimilate nutrients to be used by the body, along with flushing out wastes and toxins via the stool, urine, and sweat. Water is important to our body's ability to function so put your water bottle in the fridge and make sure you slowly get through it during the day. Benefits of keeping your water levels where they should be are a clearer mind and memory, improved digestion, improved energy and less fatigue, a decrease or elimination of headaches, less toxins in the body as water makes them more easier to be flushed out, improved skin complexion, improved bowel regularity and improved cramps or muscle spasms. So always remember water makes everything work better.

Our Diet for the Muscular Skeletal System

The best diet for this system is combining the Acid and Alkaline diet with the Mediterranean Diet which is very anti-inflammatory and also used for Cardio-vascular disease and Brain disorders such as Dementia and Alzheimer's disease. This system has some very acidy diseases with the worst being Gout where the acid gets so concentrated that it forms into crystal needle like structures that form usually in and around the big toe causing considerable pain. Another obvious one is Rheumatism which can cause deformity especially in the hands and fingers along with a lot of pain. Both of these conditions also cause a lot inflammation. These diets will be useful for people who have chronic and age related conditions and those who are athletes or do hard physical labour as the body in these conditions wears out fairly fast without you noticing, then it's too late.

The Mediterranean Diet

The Mediterranean Diet concentrates on whole grains, fresh fruits and vegetables, fish, olive oil and moderate daily Red wine consumption. This diet is not low fat. It is low in saturated fat but high in monounsaturated fat. This diet is naturally rich in fibre, antioxidants, and omega-3 fatty acids. It appears to be heart and brain healthy. With this diet you frequently hear about a long-term study of 423 people who had a heart attack, those who followed a Mediterranean style diet had a 50 to 70% lower risk of recurrent heart disease compared with people who received no dietary counselling. The reality is if you stick to this diet you are not eating processed foods loaded with saturated fat and sugars which is where most of the problem causing acids and inflammations and diseases come from. To add to this diet go through the Superfoods that follow and take what you like from them. There are lots of PDFs on the net about the **Mediterranean Diet** download about five of them so you can choose from a large variety of food that you like.

Superfoods for the Muscular Skeletal System

Apples – Apples are low in calories (90) and rich in nutrients and fibre. Apples may help due to the presence of the antioxidant quercetin that can help stabilize the cells that release histamine thereby having an anti-inflammatory and antihistamine effect. Unpeeled apples are good sources of both fibre and compounds called polyphenols that benefit heart health. The high soluble fibre in apples helps lower cholesterol, while the polyphenols lower blood pressure and stroke risk. Apples are low in calories and rich in nutrients and fibre.

Berries – Berries such as blackberries, strawberries, and blueberries are rich in Vitamin C, E, and folate which help prevent heart and many other chronic diseases and strengthen the bones and muscles. **Black Berries** - Are high in beneficial vitamins and minerals, fibre, and antioxidants. They're low in calories, carbs, and fat. One cup of raw blackberries has almost 8 grams of fibre and contains high levels of antioxidants, such as anthocyanins. Antioxidants such as anthocyanins hold many anti-inflammatory and anti-microbial properties. They may also combat diabetes and certain kinds of cancer. New research suggests that an increased intake of blackberries may address obesity by increasing insulin sensitivity and helping the body burn fat more effectively. **Raspberries** are full of fibre and antioxidant polyphenols. **Sweet Cherries** - Just 1 cup of pitted sweet cherries provides 10% of the daily dose for potassium a mineral that is essential for keeping your heart healthy. It's needed to maintain a regular heartbeat and helps remove excess sodium from your body, regulating your blood pressure. They are also rich in powerful polyphenol antioxidants, including anthocyanins, flavonols, and catechins, which may help by protecting against cellular damage and reducing inflammation. **Strawberries** are an excellent source of vitamin C. They may also help reduce risk factors for heart disease and control blood sugar. **Blueberries** - Are one of the highest berries in antioxidants. The dark blue pigment found in blueberries contains phenols called anthocyanins which are flavonoids with powerful antioxidant capabilities that have been shown to protect tissue from oxidative damage. Blueberries are high in nitric oxide, a molecule that relaxes the inner muscles of blood vessels. This characteristic helps lower blood pressure and slows the aging of the blood vessel. They also are a significant source of vitamin C, manganese and are high in soluble fibre which helps your gut remove bile and manage cholesterol; it does this by binding to the cholesterol, salts, minerals, and other bile components and removing it through the body's waste. Good for your eyes to. This fruit may help protect the brain from the damage caused by free radicals and may reduce the effects of age-related conditions such as Alzheimer's or dementia.

Broccoli - Broccoli contains a number of compounds that have powerful antioxidant and anti-inflammatory effects which can help with premature ageing and inflammatory conditions.

Broccoli is a superfood because it contains both glucosinolates and large amounts of other nutrients such as calcium, vitamins A, B, C and K, beta-carotene, iron and fibre. These nutrients protect against free radicals, keep blood flowing well, and can remove heavy metals. Broccoli is rich with vitamin K and calcium, which are two nutrients that are important for healthy bones and joints. Add broccoli to you diet four times each week. **Warning** – Too much Broccoli can give you wind.

Eggs - A boiled egg will have more benefits to health than an omelet or other forms. Besides being rich in proteins, eggs contain essential nutrients and minerals such as vitamin D, Omega 3 fatty acids and folate. The list of its nutritional prowess seems endless, but in reality it is obvious as its main reason for being is to create life so it has to have everything inside that is needed. Eggs have in them a very important micronutrient that your body needs called Choline which is used to create acetylcholine which is an neurotransmitter that helps regulate mood and memory and is also used for conditions such as Alzheimer's and Huntington's disease, memory problems and depression. Eggs benefits to bone health are vitamin D, zinc and the osteogenic bioactive components lutein and zeaxanthin. One egg gives you a quarter of the daily dose. It also helps with blood pressure and hardening of the arteries. Eggs are also a good supply of selenium, vitamins A, E, B2, B5, B12, as well as iron, iodine and phosphorus.

Ginger - Ginger has been a part of cooking and traditional medicine for thousands of years. Some of gingers health benefits may be attributed to its digestive enzymes but here we will be using it for its strong anti-inflammatory action in rheumatism, osteoarthritis and joint injuries. Ginger contains the digestive enzyme zingibain, which is a protease that digests proteins. It may aid digestion by helping food move faster through the digestive tract and boosting the body's own production of digestive enzymes. Studies in healthy adults and those with indigestion, show that ginger helps food move faster through the stomach by promoting contractions. Ginger is rich in vitamins C, B complex, copper, potassium, calcium, zinc, magnesium and manganese and helps promote circulation, stimulates digestion, alleviates nausea and has anti-inflammatory and antioxidant properties.

Oats and Oatmeal – This wholegrain is full of soluble fibre which prevents the body from absorbing cholesterol. Beta-glucan fibre in oats is effective at reducing both total and LDL cholesterol levels and may increase the release of cholesterol rich bile from the liver. The antioxidants in oats also have anti-inflammatory properties which can help reducing inflammation in the arteries and anywhere else in the body. Body builders like it because it increases bone stamina. Oats are high in calcium, copper, zinc and magnesium which are good for increasing bone density. Rolled oats are good but steel cut oats are better as they have more fibre and the fibre is denser.

Olive Oil Extra Virgin – Consuming more than half a table spoon of olive oil a day may lower the heart disease risk a 2020 study found. Olive oil is one of the key components of the Mediterranean diet which is well known for its heart health. Olive oil is rich in monounsaturated fat which helps lower the harmful LDL cholesterol. When olive oil replaces saturated fat like butter it can help lower cholesterol levels. As the oil was cold pressed without heat and chemicals all the polyphenols where saved. The natural compound oleocanthal blocks the same inflammatory pathways as certain NSAIDs. Additionally, the polyphenol extract found in extra virgin olive oil can decrease joint oedema, cell migration, cartilage degradation, and bone erosion. The oil also contains Omega 3 fats that help to train and maintain the muscles. This is especially important for an athlete who is exposed to significant wear and tear. Olive oil in its natural state significantly decreases arthritis pain and inflammatory symptoms.

Prunes – Prunes are actually dried plums and are rich in fibre, antioxidants, vitamins and minerals. They are good for weight because they contain pectin which acts as a natural laxative to remove waste from your body fairly fast which is why they are used for constipation. One of the reason I have added prunes is that they are now being used to help against Osteoporosis and Osteopenia, after a clinical study showed that dried plums may be able to reverse osteoporosis in post-menopausal women. The women that were asked to eat 100 grams of prunes per day had improved bone formation markers after only three months, compared to a control group who were eating 75 grams of dried apples. The health benefits of prunes may be linked to their high concentration of the trace element boron which is meant to play a role in prevention (boron hardens the surface of bone) of osteoporosis and osteopenia. This may also be due to the high levels of vitamin K in prunes. Prune consumption preserves bone mass density and strength at weight-bearing sites in the hip. Women who did not eat prunes saw a 1.1% decrease in bone density, while women who ate five or six prunes each day experienced no measurable loss of bone density. Eating 5 to 6 prunes a day may prevent bone loss. Prunes are a good source of beta carotene which the body converts to vitamin A. Others are vitamin K, potassium, zinc, iron, calcium, magnesium, manganese, copper, and B vitamins.

Salmon and Fatty Fish - What makes oily fish so good is that they contain active fats in a ready-made form which means the body can use it easily. Essential fatty acids (EFAs) cannot be made by the body so they must be obtained through our diet. The most effective one omega-3 fats occur naturally in oily fish in the form of EPA and

DHA. A diet with higher levels of these fats may help in lowering the risks of dementia and also slows mental decline as well as helping heart and circulation and toning down inflammatory responses. Salmon, trout, tuna, herring and sardines are all good rich sources. About 60% of your brain is made of fat, and half of that fat is comprised of omega-3 fatty acids. Your brain uses omega 3 to build brain and nerve cells and these fats are essential for learning and the memory. For brain health two servings of fish per week are recommended. Fish oil is good for other inflammatory diseases such as Rheumatism and Arthritis. Fish with the highest amount of these good oils always live in the coldest waters. If you don't like fish you could invest in some Fish Oil Capsules the EPA and DHA content should be written on the label. An 85 gram serving of canned salmon has 180 mg of calcium. It's rich in the calcium because the can contains the tiny soft bones which have been cooked in the can. It's the same for Sardines which is why they are high in calcium.

Sardines Canned – A can of sardines is full of everything. When you eat fish along with the bones and skin you are getting most of what our body requires for a health. A 105 gram can of sardines has approximately 350 mg of calcium and 178 IUs of vitamin D, which is about one-third and one-half of the daily requirements for people over 50, vitamin D allows your body to absorb calcium. Sardines also contain omega-3 fatty acids, proteins, B12, nutrients, and other mineral supplements. Sardines also contain another bone boosting nutrient which is phosphorous.

Sesame Seeds – Small amounts only maybe every day, consider it a micro-nutrient. Have potent anti-inflammatory properties that help keep the inflammatory processes toned down in your body. They are also an excellent source of Manganese and Calcium, both of which help your bones grow healthy and strong. They also contain Zinc, Magnesium, Iron, Molybdenum, Selenium and B1. You can use them as seeds which you would have seen as the black seeds on some bread and also as oil, milk and flour. **Cautions** – Only use small quantities of Sesame as they can lower blood sugar and drop blood pressure in large quantities. People with Gout should avoid them as they contain Oxalates which are a natural substance that causes aggravation of gout symptoms. People with allergies should also be careful.

Turmeric – Has the medical action of an anti-inflammatory, anti-oxidant, anti-cancer, anti-biotic and microbial, circulatory stimulant, alterative, liver restorative and protector.

This was kind of the forgotten herb that has now rocketed on to the market. I think most of the old Western Herbalists decided they would just use Ginger as Turmeric comes from the same family. This herb is a main arthritis remedy where it is very helpful with pain relief due to its powerful anti-inflammatory effects, so it will help with Rheumatism to. Used also in Tendonitis, Bursitis and generally for any pain accompanied by inflammation. It is rich in vitamins, calcium, and other important minerals. So add this herb in a really big container to your spice shelf.

Walnuts – These nuts are packed with omega 3s the healthy monosaturated fats, plant sterols and fibre. A small handful of walnuts a day can lower your cholesterol and help reduce inflammatory problems in the arteries. Eating walnuts can reduce the risk of developing osteoporosis especially in the aged. The magnesium found in walnuts can help seniors maintain bone strength and slow down bone loss. Magnesium is important for bone formation as it helps with the absorption of calcium into the bone. High in unsaturated omega-3 fatty acids, iron and B vitamins walnuts have powerful antioxidant properties which makes them beneficial to whole-body health.

Yogurt Plain – Is high in Calcium with a small cup giving you about 250 mg of calcium and you can add it to anything you want and flavour it anyway you want. It also contains vitamins A, D, and B 12. Bones will improve their stamina and become strong if eaten every day.

Whole Grains – People especially those that are underweight need to be built up again, with the best way being to supply this energy by choosing whole grains which give a slow sugar release into the bloodstream. White bread, white sugar and other refined sugars give a far too big rush of sugar which overwhelms the body loading it with acid and eventually leading to diabetes. Too much sugar flowing through the arteries along with the wrong types and unnatural fats damages the whole system especially the arteries and prematurely ages the whole body. The slow release of sugars by whole meal and grain products keeps our bodies supplied throughout the day. Whole grains also provide a wide range of nutrients and antioxidants. Whole-grain foods are brown rice, barley, bulgur wheat, oatmeal, millet, whole-grain bread and whole-grain pasta. Carbs are often considered the enemy when it comes to health, but whole grains are rich in complex carbohydrates, fibre, and some omega-3 fatty acids that shield the heart and brain from damaging sugar spikes, cholesterol, blood clots, and more. Grains also contain B vitamins that have an effect on blood flow to the brain and mood. Whole grains should be soaked, fermented, sprouted, or grown as sprouts to unlock all their nutritional power.

Osteoporosis and Bone Pains

This disorder is characterized by a slow and progressive thinning and loss of the calcium content of the bones along with other minerals. Although the process actually begins in the fourth decade in both sexes it is accelerated in women after menopause. We all know the nasty things that can happen like hip fractures etc etc so I won't go into details. The first early warning signs of osteoporosis are those of calcium deficiency such as nocturnal leg cramps, joint pain, transparent skin, restless behavior and insomnia. In severe cases symptoms are a very painful backache especially in the upper back. Always remember prevention is much easier then cure. Some medications interfere with calcium absorption; the ones to be weary of and to ask your pharmacist about are Corticosteroids, Anticonvulsants, Antacids containing aluminum and some Diuretics. The book has an Acid and Alkaline Chart for the reason that excessively acid bodies try to make themselves more Alkaline so they tend to use what is easily available to do this which is usually Calcium and Magnesium which do a good job of buffering acid. Too much protein puts acid in the system, mainly uric acid which results from the breakdown of protein. Sugar put lots of acid in the body along with alcohol which when you break it down is just sugar.

Disease and Cancer are found in Acid bodies, it is said Cancer can't live in an Alkaline body. Use alkaline foods to correct the imbalance. This is what the chart is for, it allows you to see if your diet is to acid and it shows you how to change it by eating more alkaline foods and reducing the acid foods.

High Risk Factors for Osteoporosis

1. A diet high in animal protein
2. Women who are light boned.
3. Women who don't take enough exercise.
4. People who have been on lots of punishing diets.
5. Women who smoke as this brings on menopause earlier.
6. Women who have a genetic predisposition to it i.e. mother had it.
7. Poor unbalanced diet.
8. Caffeine and alcohol encourage the excretion of calcium.
9. Excessive salt intake makes our bodies excrete calcium and phosphorus.
10. Certain drugs increase the risk of osteoporosis examples are cortisone, thyroxine, tamoxifen, diuretics and antacids.
11. Women who have had total hysterectomies including removal of their ovaries.
12. Being underweight.
13. Poor absorption of nutrients by the digestive system.

Nutrition for Osteoporosis and the Bones

Calcium supplements are often poorly absorbed especially inorganic sources such as dolomite. Calcium should be combined with magnesium in the ratio of 2 to 1. A supplement should ideally contain other minerals and vitamins needed in the right proportions. Calcium taken alone depletes zinc and iron. Try a supplement that goes something like this 1000mg calcium, 500mg magnesium, 10mg zinc, 3mg boron and a bit of Vitamin D. Take with it about 1000mg of vitamin C daily. Even better try to get your calcium and minerals naturally from the diet, the only problem here is that only about 20 to 40% of calcium is absorbed and this gets worse with age. Vitamin D is needed for the absorption of calcium and for the body to make vitamin D it needs exposure to sunlight so make sure you get a bit of sun every day, go for a walk and strengthen your bones. Milk and other dairy products are not necessarily the best sources for natural calcium. Milk is low in magnesium which is needed to assimilate calcium and there are other foods that are higher. The table below suggests some other sources.

Boron - Boron is required for strong bones and the full absorption of calcium. Sources are apples, pears, grapes, dates, raisins, peaches, soybeans, almonds, hazelnuts, peanuts and honey. As a micro nutrient the dose is small about 1 to 2mg a day so a good dose is 2 apples and 3 and a half ounces of peanuts.

Calcium Rich Foods

Kelp (sea weed) per 100 grams	1093mg
Blackstrap molasses per 100 grams	579mg
Sardines per 100 grams	550mg
Dried figs per 100 grams	280mg
Almonds per 100 grams	250mg
Watercress per 100 grams	220mg
Sunflower seeds per 100 grams	100mg
Tofu per 100 grams	128mg

Comparison with Dairy Foods

Tofu per 100 grams	120mg
Cheddar Cheese per 50 grams	400mg
Yogurt per 100 grams	180mg

The Main Nutrition for Muscles

This is similar to what the bones like but if you are giving your muscles a hard time through sport or hard physical labour you must ensure you keep the body hydrated and that you are having adequate protein so as to repair the damage you are doing to the muscles. Staying hydrated supports digestion and nutrient absorption and transportation. Thick blood has a hard time getting into little blood vessels.

Protein - Protein is one of the most essential macronutrients for muscle growth and repair and also in the whole body itself, for amino acids are the body's building blocks. Signs of deficiency can be brittle hair and nails, muscle weakness, stress fractures, feeling weak or hungry. **Protein Sources** are Dairy foods, meat, seafood's, eggs, beans and other legumes and Soy.

Calcium - Builds strong bones and prevents osteoporosis but also does a lot more. In an average human body there is about 1 kg of calcium of which 99% is in the bones. The last one percent is used mostly in the nerves, muscles and also for buffering high acid levels in the body so as to keep the blood slightly alkaline. Your body needs calcium for muscles to move and for nerves to carry messages between your brain and every part of your body and where would your teeth be without it. The bones act as a store house for calcium and allows the blood which is the main transport system, to take what is needed to other parts of the body. Calcium is one of the main building blocks of life. People with Crohn's or Coeliac disease will have problems absorbing calcium along with those who are lactose intolerant. **Calcium Sources** – Yogurt, fortified milk, almond milk, cheese, tofu, green leafy vegetables, salmon, sardines and whey.

Magnesium – This mineral is what the nerves and muscles run on so any deficiency here you will know fairly fast usually in the manner of cramps or tiredness. Stress and worry is one of the main culprits as it never rests. A good fast cure is Chamomile tea as it is loaded with calcium and magnesium as they are buddies and like to hang out together. **Magnesium Sources** – Chamomile tea, if you don't like it just add a Peppermint tea bag and you will forget about the Chamomile. Other sources are green leafy vegetables, spinach, beans, cashews, nuts and seeds, wholegrains, brown rice, bananas and oatmeal, maybe have a nice porridge.

Glutamine – Glutamine helps repair muscle and tissues. Glutamine is an amino acid produced by the body and found in food. It also supports your body's immune and digestive systems. Injuries can be a cause of the body becoming deficient. **Glutamine Sources** – As it is an amino acid it will be found in protein so good sources of it are chicken, fish, beef, pork, dairy foods, eggs, cheese, cottage cheese, spinach and red cabbage.

Vitamin D - Vitamin D is linked to healthy hormones like testosterone which helps with muscle maintenance and growth and can also improve your mental health and help reduce anxiety. Vitamin D is needed for the absorption of calcium and for the body to make vitamin D it also needs exposure to sunlight, so make sure you get a bit of sun every day, go for a walk and strengthen your bones. Lack of this vitamin causes Rickets in children and softening of the bones. **Vitamin D Sources -** Fatty fish, like salmon and sardines, fortified yogurt, milk and orange juice, mushrooms and eggs.

Gout Diet

Gout is a painful form of arthritis that is associated with elevated levels of uric acid in the blood. High levels of uric acid can cause crystals to form in the joints and especially in the big toe with this condition causing pain and swelling and in the past when not much was known about diets, it caused severe pain and misery and was a condition found in the rich. We now know that the main culprit for this condition is from the breakdown of food compounds called purines. It is now believed that lowering uric acid levels through changes in your diet may help reduce future attacks. Purines are a type of protein found in many foods and are in all of your cells. It is advised to act quickly to resolve this condition as it can cause damage to the kidneys and other problems like type two diabetes. Half of people with Gout are overweight so this has to be also dealt with but it is a good way to begin treatment for it starts to reduce the uric acid in the blood very quickly, which will then reduce the attacks. Uric acid is made in the body from the breakdown of purines that come from your diet so you need to take control of your diet and avoid foods high in Purines.

High Purine Foods to Avoid

Offal - Liver and kidneys, heart and sweetbreads.

Game Meat - Pheasant, rabbit, venison.

Oily Fish - Anchovies, herring, mackerel, sardines, sprats, whitebait, trout.

Seafood - Mussels, crab, shrimps and other shellfish, fish, roe, caviar.

Meat and Yeast Extracts - Marmite, Promite, Bovril, commercial gravy as well as beer.

Moderate Purine Foods (Take in Moderation)

Meat - Beef, lamb chicken, pork.

Poultry - Chicken and duck

Dried peas, beans and legumes - Baked beans, kidney beans, soya beans and peas etc.

Vegetables - Asparagus, cauliflower, spinach.

Wholegrains - Bran, oatbran, wholemeal bread.

Low Purine Foods

Dairy - milk, cheese, yoghurt, butter.

Breads and cereals – Except wholegrain.

Pasta and Noodles

Fruit and Vegetables

Eggs

Alcohol - Alcohol can increase your risk of developing gout and can bring on a sudden attack if you are already a gout sufferer. Alcohol can raise uric acid levels in the blood and trigger a gout attack. Many beers contain large quantities of purines from the fermenting process and alcohol stimulates the production of uric acid by the liver. Champagne, Red wine and Port may be worse than other forms of alcohol but all types have an effect.

Weight Lose - Being overweight can cause an increase in uric acid and puts more strain on the joints and kidneys. Try to reduce your intake of high energy foods such as fats and sugars. Forget about the fast diets as you may get into trouble as strict dieting can bring on an attack of gout by loading up the body with acid. Slowly but surely is the way to go, but also find foods that you like that are good for you.

Water - Drinking water reduces the likelihood of crystals forming in the kidneys. As a general rule, drinking 8 large glasses of fluids a day (1.5 litres) is recommended. It is best to use water as it dilutes the system and takes out more rubbish then it puts in.

Vitamin C - Some studies have shown that a diet high in vitamin C may prevent Gout. Vitamin C used as a dietary supplement at about 500 to 1500mg throughout the day can reduce blood uric acid levels. A study of almost 47,000 men over a 20-year period found that those taking a vitamin C supplement had a 44 percent lower gout risk.

Fibromyalgia Diet

There is no Fibromyalgia diet but if there was one it would be very similar to the Mediterranean Diet which we are using for the Muscular Skeletal System. The Mediterranean Diet **Limits saturated**

fat and trans-fat. You need some saturated fat but only in small amounts. Eating too much saturated fat can raise your bad cholesterol. Trans-fat has no health benefits and can cause inflammation. The Mediterranean Diet **encourages healthy unsaturated fats especially omega-3 fatty acids.** Unsaturated fats promote healthy cholesterol levels and combat inflammation and also promote healthy blood sugar levels. Talking about sugar, this diet **limits refined carbohydrates, including sugar.** Foods high in refined carbs can cause your blood sugar to spike which forces the body to do a big squirt of insulin to get them down. Refined carbs also give you excess calories without much or any nutritional benefit. The Mediterranean Diet **favours foods high in fibre and antioxidants.** These nutrients again help reduce inflammation throughout your body. Fibre keeps the waste moving through your large intestine and reduces constipation. **It is best to consider Fibromyalgia as a kind of autoimmune disease such as a mild kind of Asthma, allergy type of fault in the autoimmune system, especially if you have the Chronic Fatigue type or the sleep and IBS type.** Always pay attention and look out for what could be an autoimmune response causing more severity and sensitivity then there should be. Antioxidants protect your cells form free radical attacks that damage cells and cause inflammation, so here you are taking your attack on the immune system to the cellular level. Vitamin C can help tone down nasty autoimmune responses and is a valuable tool if your suspicion of an autoimmune problem is found to be true. And finally this diet **limits sodium**. A diet high in sodium can raise your blood pressure putting you at greater risk for a heart attack or stroke. **Being overweight** can worsen autoimmune problems so eat to maintain a healthy weight. If you are overweight start to slowly loose it, as even losing a little weight can improve your symptoms and fast diets seem to always have a rebound affect. So work out a diet that you can live with and slowly get to your right weight. Next learn how to eat to maintain a healthy weight over the long term by eating plenty of fruits and vegetables as they're a good source of antioxidants, such as beta carotene used to make vitamin A and vitamins C and E, which may help reduce lung swelling and inflammation caused by cell-damaging chemicals known as free radicals. **Be careful with allergy-triggering foods (get an allergy test to be safe)** such as milk, eggs, peanuts and some sea foods such as prawns and shell fish. Allergic food reactions can cause autoimmune problems in some people and this is important to get checked in Fibromyalgia as it could be a cause of lots of other problems to.

Avoid sulphites as they can trigger autoimmune symptoms in some people. Sulphites used as a preservative can be found in wine, dried fruits, pickles, fresh and frozen shrimp and some other foods. I would also be inclined to avoid foods with lots of nitrates in them such as processed meats. Be careful of **artificial ingredients** such as chemical preservatives, flavourings, and colourings that are often found in processed and fast food. Some people with autoimmune problems may be sensitive or allergic to these artificial ingredients. **Salicylate sensitivity** is common in 5 to 20% of asthmatics who are hypersensitive to aspirin and many fruits and some vegetables that contain salicylates. Foods that contain are Broccoli, cauliflower, cucumber, mushrooms, radishes, spinach and zucchini all contain high amounts of salicylates. Vegetables from the nightshade family, like eggplant and peppers, also contain salicylates. Tomatoes are very high in salicylates. To end here consider a Mediterranean Diet minis what can cause you problems, as you need to know your dangers and add in other foods that you like that are healthy, then take it from there and see what happens.

Vitamin C – Most Important for Allergies and Auto-immunes Problems

Vitamin C is the most critical supplement for the natural treatment of Autoimmune Problems as it is the primary antioxidant in the lungs and a powerful antihistamine without side effects. Low vitamin C dramatically increases histamine levels which put you at greater risk for allergic reactions, rhinitis, and asthma attacks. 1000mg of C for three days reduces blood histamine to normal levels. Vitamin C reduces the severity of allergic responses but be aware that your body gobbles up C during prolonged asthma or allergy attacks and if it is not replaced the attacks may get worse and worse. Vitamin C is needed by the immune system and is necessary for healing and the prevention of infections along with being a potent antioxidant with anti-bacterial and antiviral actions. Alleviates asthma by inhibiting the bronchial constriction that occurs during asthma attacks and by helping reduce the excessive histamine levels that commonly occur in people affected with asthma. Humans do not manufacture Vitamin C and neither is it stored by the body so the diet is the only source. Vitamin C is easily depleted in the body especially by smoking (25mg per cigarette), stress, pollution and alcohol. Always remember to increase the dose to the severity of the attack. A good preventative dose for adults would be to take 1000mg three times per day eg breakfast, lunch and tea so that there is always a good amount in the body to be drawn upon. In acute conditions or in pollen season think about taking 1000mg every 3 to 4 hours. Always have a big bottle of vitamin C ready.

Zinc - Most people these days are deficient in zinc which is required by the immune system for optimum function and healing. Zinc can be deficient in a person with chronic allergies. Normal levels of zinc in the blood stream inhibit the release of histamine from mast cells and low levels of zinc are associated with chemical sensitivities. Zinc is also a potent antioxidant and if you are taking a good antioxidant formula zinc should be in it. One of the richest sources of zinc are oysters, other sources are liver, meat, seeds, green leafy vegetables and whole grains. **Dose** - 10 to 40mg per day depending on severity.

Exercise - Low-intensity exercise is one of the most effective treatments for fibromyalgia. At first you may experience a slight increase in pain and soreness when you start, which is normal, but as you continue you will help lessen muscle tension and stiffness, improve sleep quality, and raise serotonin and endorphin levels which help to reduce pain. The old saying, Use it or Loose it has a lot of truth in it.

Our Main Supplement for Joint Injuries
Glucosamine Sulphate, Chondroitin Sulphate and (MSM) Formula

I have been using this formula and very similar to this for over 30 years. In my youth I wore my back out in the Heavy Transport industry after lifting 30 Tons a day for years loading specialized containers, train wagons along with driving fork lifts in the latter half of the day, loading after all the sorting out and grouping was finished. Getting towards the end I was living on this formula. Half way through the day and in the evening and first thing in the morning I would take my oversized scoop and mix it with water, then wait 20 minutes and jump up and grab my metal bar which hung from the roof rafters. I would hang there as long as I could, for I was putting my back in traction and as all the cartilage between the disks in the back were pulled apart it would suck in the formula and I could continue for another day. Unfortunately you can only do this for so long, well nearly a decade for me on and off. Over time I learnt the value of this formula in first aid, in sprains and strains and generally in any tissue damage in the joints. I have also used the formula on animals during the times I have worked on farms especially in the tropics of Australia. I know of those who use it for race horses as it really annoyed me, as I usually buy it in 1 kg tubs and he was buying it in 20 litre buckets for only a little more than I was paying with the only difference being the bucket said not fit for humans which was probably a lie, as you would be very weary of what you would give a million dollar race horse. I still use the formula today; it sits there waiting for me to do something stupid. The Ingredients of the formula follow.

Glucosamine Sulphate - Has many biological functions among which are its role as a stimulant and precursor to the proteins that form cartilage. As we age our ability to produce GS decreases and causes the cartilage to lose its water holding capability causing the cartilage to become dry and ineffective as a shock absorber, leading to pain. GS normalizes cartilage metabolism and prevents cartilage degradation. Stimulates the biosynthesis of the key structural components of cartilage (mucopolysaccharides) that are essential for healthy joint function and repair. Mucopolysaccharides also allow the cartilage to hold water which in turn acts as a shock absorber. GS also acts as a mild anti-inflammatory and combines with **Chondroitin** for effective joint repair and helps relieve the pain and inflammation of arthritis and joint injuries. Beneficial to athletes affected by cartilage or joint problems and halts cartilage destruction and encourages the regeneration of new cartilage.

Chondroitin Sulphate - Occurs naturally in the cartilage where it participates in the matrix structure. CS protects cartilage from degradation by inhibiting elastase which is the enzyme responsible for the degradation of cartilage and increases the synthesis of proteoglycans which is a key structural component of cartilage. Together with GS, CS has been found to increase hyaluronate concentration and viscosity of synovial fluid increasing lubrication within the joints. Like GS, CS exerts only a mild anti-inflammatory action and for this reason both are usually given together with anti-inflammatory nutrients such as MSM and bioflavonoids in order to obtain faster pain relief. Vitamins C, E, B3, B5, and B6 are also valuable adjuncts to supplementation with GS and CS.

Methyl Sulfonyl Methane (MSM) - Is a naturally occurring source of organic Sulphur. The concentration of Sulphur in arthritic cartilage has been shown to be about one third the level of normal cartilage. Other beneficial effects of MSM are due to its ability to reduce inflammation and to inhibit pain impulses along nerve fibers. Can be of benefit in conditions of bursitis, tendonitis, tennis elbow and RSI.

As we age the levels of MSM in the body decrease.

Nutralife Joint Formula + MSM Lemon Powder
(Taken from a ebay sale write-up)

This is fairly much the same as the formula I have been taking now for more the 30 years. I recently had to purchase some more so I decided to get a big 1 kg size and found it on ebay. Below is a straight copy form the sales pitch.

Benefits & Features

Scientifically formulated Nutra-Life Joint Formula + MSM powder combines MSM with Glucosamine sulfate and Chondroitin sulfate, both of which have been shown to support the health and function of joints. Also included are important supporting nutrients – Copper and Manganese to help maintain connective tissue. Glucosamine is produced naturally in the body where it is important for maintaining the elasticity, strength and resilience of cartilage in joints. Glucosamine is also a key building block for cartilage, tendons, ligaments and synovial fluid while Chondroitin supports the health and function of the joints. MSM is a source of sulfur. Cartilage has a high content of sulfur and is required for the formation of connective tissue.

When taken regularly, Nutra-Life Joint Formula + MSM powder may help:

- Support healthy joint function
- Support the development and maintenance of cartilage
- Assist with healthy joint mobility

AVAILABLE IN 500G and 1KG

Always read the label and follow the directions for use. Please read the dosages & warnings information before purchase

Ingredients

Serving size 15g (1 level scoop) Serves per day: 2 level scoops (30g). Servings per 1kg pack = 66. Per 15g Per 30g (daily dose)

Contains

- Bovine sodium chondroitin sulfate 682mg 1.36g
- Equiv. Chondroitin sulfate 600mg 1.2g
- Dimethyl sulfone (MSM) 750mg 1.5g

- Glucosamine sulfate potassium chloride 750mg 1.5g
- Equiv. Glucosamine sulfate 565mg 1.13g
- Equiv. Potassium chloride 185mg 370mg
- Cofactors
- Ascorbic acid (Vitamin C) 150mg 300mg
- Boron (as Borax) 500µg 1000µg
- Copper (as gluconate) 500µg 1000µg
- Manganese (as sulfate monohydrate) 3mg 6mg
- Zinc (as oxide) 6mg 12mg
- Glucose
- Maltodextrin
- Natural flavours
- Silicon dioxide

Formulated without - Gluten, wheat, dairy products, egg, soy, artificial colours, artificial flavours or artificial sweeteners. Always read the label. Use only as directed. If symptoms persist, consult your health professional.

Dosage & Warnings

Recommended Adult Dosage: Add 1 level scoop (15g) to 250mL water or fruit juice twice daily. Mix thoroughly prior to consumption and take with meals. Alternatively 1 level scoop (15g) can be added to food twice daily. Or as directed by your healthcare professional.

Warnings - Always read the label and follow directions for use. Contains 97mg of Potassium per 15g serve. If you have kidney disease or are taking heart or blood pressure medicines, consult your doctor or pharmacist before use. DERIVED FROM SEAFOOD.

Herbal for the Muscular Skeletal System
Astragalus
Astragalus membranaceus

Actions - Immuno-modulator, anti-viral, adaptogen, hypotensive, immune stimulant, adrenal tonic, diuretic, vasodilator, cardiotonic, antioxidant, hepatoprotective, hypoglycemic.

This herb should only be used in chronic diseases, as a preventative or in cases of fatigue especially in chronic diseases. Stimulates the natural production of interferon and intensifies the white cell destruction of germs. A good tonic for strengthening the resistance to disease. Is very useful for chronic debility and fatigue by restoring the immune function. Use as a lung tonic to help expel toxins and pus in flu's, colds and sinusitis. Increases stamina and can accelerate wound healing, can help to replenish bone marrow. Strengthens the digestive system and aids adrenal gland function. This herb is used for cancer especially if the patient has had chemotherapy and helps aid them in their recovery. Thought to control body fluids such as excessive sweating, night sweats and relieve fluid retention. Astragalus has powerful anti-aging properties slowing the aging process at a cellular level. Astragaloside IV a saponin has shown benefits in reversing cell damage and in activating telomerase, this addresses telomere shortening and slows down cellular aging. This is very important, I will try to explain. Inside every cell of your body is a Telomere, a good way to think about it is as an hour glass. Every time a cell divides it breaks a little piece of the telomere off which is a bit of sand flowing through the hour glass, when the last piece of the telomere is gone that is the last time the cell can divide, this is how we age. Now I will explain why Antioxidants are so important. Imagine a nasty little free radical with a baseball bat which has just smashed into one of your cells and is wandering round inside your cell and then comes across the telomere and says I will fix you and smashes the telomere right at the bottom and leaves only a little stump left. That's it for the cell, his life has been cut short. Astragalus root is most effective when taken long term, providing many benefits that can contribute to a longer, healthier life. Good to use for chronic fatigue syndrome (CFS) and fibromyalgia. Has cardioprotective effects helping to prevent plaque buildup in the arteries and narrowing of the blood vessel walls by protecting the inner wall of the vessel. It has also been shown to reduce blood pressure and lower triglycerides. **Immune Boosting -** Is an immune stimulant that is known to increase the count of white blood cells and stimulate the production of antibodies, this builds up bodily resistance to viruses and bacteria. Many clinical studies have shown it boosts the immune system and encourages an increase in immune T-cells, natural killer cells, macrophages and immunoglobulin activity, production and function. Astragalus appears to trigger immune cells from a resting state into heightened activity. The natural killer cells of the immune system also seem to be markedly enhanced to fight intruders five to six times higher than normal. **Cautions** - Should not be used in acute infections or fevers. Use with care for those with very low blood pressure. Women who are pregnant or breastfeeding should not use Astragalus. May counteract anti-diabetic agents and potentiate effects of diuretics. People with autoimmune diseases should consult their healthcare professional before using Astragalus because of its ability to stimulate the immune system. **Part used –** Root. **Dose** - 500 to a 1000mg per day or up to 20 drops of tincture twice daily.

Boswellia

Frankincense

Actions – Anti-inflammatory, anti-arthritic, analgesic, ant rheumatic, liver protective.

A traditional remedy for wound healing and inflammatory diseases that has been used in many cultures. Also used for respiratory diseases especially the chronic ones and rheumatic disorders, diarrhoea, dysentery, piles, dysmenorrhoea and in weakness to improve the appetite and liver disorders. Studies have shown that the essential oil provides immune stimulant activity throughout the body with one study finding that Frankincense increases white blood cell production whilst keeping inflammation at a minimum. When applied topically, the oil will work to create a layer of protection against bacterial and viral infections. When inhaled the same benefits manifest internally working to heal the body from the inside out. In arthritis and rheumatism its powerful anti-inflammatory compounds such as terpenes and boswellic acids reduce joint inflammation by preventing the release of leukotrienes that can cause inflammation, with studies confirming it may be as effective as NSAIDS with no negative side effects. Frankincense essential oil can be massaged into painful joints and muscles, and has been found useful in preventing the breakdown of cartilage tissue, thus reducing inflammation. **Frankincense Essential Oil** - Frankincense essential oil is able to rejuvenate and revive tired skin and as such it is added to many beautifying lotions. Frankincense essential oil can be used in the bath, or vaporized in an oil burner. It can be added to a massage oil or cream. Use 6 to 8 drops per bath and 10 to 18 drops per 30ml of carrier oil. **Constituents -** The major constituents of Frankincense are acid resins, gum, 3-acetyl-beta-boswellic acid, alpha-boswellic acid, methyl-glucuronic acid, incensole acetate, terpines, phellandrene and pentacyclic triterpenoids. **Precautions -** None known. **Dose –** Tincture - 1 to 3 ml three times a day. Capsules 300 to 400 mg three times a day or as labelled.

Cats Claw

Uncaria tomentosa

Actions - Anti oxidant, immune stimulant, anti-inflammatory, anti-fungal, anti-rheumatic, anti-viral, anti-tumor, hypotensive, anti-microbial.

Primary traditional uses in Peru are as an anti-inflammatory, contraceptive and anti-cancer remedy. An immune stimulant especially used in viral infections, including HIV. Useful in a variety of inflammatory diseases including gastric ulcers, diarrhea and GI tumors, gonorrhea, arthritis and rheumatism, acne, diabetes, diseases of the urinary tract and cancer. Also used to alleviate allergic sinus type conditions, boost the immune system, asthma, bursitis, Candida, immune deficiency disorders, chronic inflammatory diseases with auto immune conditions. With a lengthy history dating back to the Inca civilization, Cat's Claw has been used as a traditional medicine in the Andes to treat inflammation, gastric ulcers, rheumatism, dysentery, intestinal complaints and wounds. **Immune System** - A recent study showed that Cat's Claw significantly elevated the infection fighting white blood cell count in adult men who supplemented with this herb for 6 months. Researchers also noted a repair in DNA – both single and double strand breaks. Its effect on the immune system appears to be two fold, with the ability to both boost and dampen immune response, depending on what is needed. Hyper immune responses can be contained, whilst a weak immune system is strengthened by supplementation with Cat's Claw. **Arthritis Relief -** Multiple studies have found that Cat's Claw can be used to naturally improve osteoarthritis and rheumatoid arthritis symptoms. In a 2001 study they found that pain associated with activity were significantly reduced within the first week of therapy. Another study noted that treatment with Cat's Claw extract resulted in a reduction in the number of painful joints compared with the placebo after 24 weeks of treatment. This arthritis fighting effect is thought to be from compounds that seem to be immune system modulators. **Constituents** - Cats Claw has many phytochemical elements that consist of oxidole alkaloids, quinovic acid glycosides, antioxidants, plant sterols and carboxyl alkyl esters. All of these are thought to have, in varying degrees, an action that can be attributed to the many benefits of Cats Claw. **Dose** - As labeled by supplier. **Parts used** - Inner bark of roots and stems. The bark is considered to be the most medicinally useful. Both Leaves and roots have been proven to hold significant phytochemical content but not in such concentration as is found in the bark. Traditionally the bark of Cats Claw is made into a tea or powder to be consumed over a given period depending on illness. **Contraindications** - Pregnancy, lactation or in children less than three years old. **Interactions** - Typically not recommended for those taking insulin, thymus extracts, vaccines, immune globulin or sera. **Precautions** - Do not take Cat's Claw if on blood thinning medication. Large quantities can cause stomach upset because of the large number of tannins in the bark. It is recommended to increase dose in increments to lessen the symptoms of detoxification. Not recommended to take Cat's Claw if you are going to have surgery.

Celery Seed
Apium graveolens

Actions - Anti-inflammatory, antimicrobial, anti-rheumatic, bitter, carminative, hypotensive, antispasmodic, diuretic, sedative.

Celery seeds are rich in powerful diuretic oils that cleanse the body of excess fluids and stimulate the kidneys to flush out uric acid and excess crystals that can cause many problems such as gout, arthritis and kidney stones. Detoxes the musculoskeletal system and used in the elimination of uric acid and waste products and also as a urinary antiseptic. It can also be useful in nervous restlessness and spasmodic tension. You can also use Celery Seed to help lower your blood pressure as it acts both as a diuretic and a vasodilator working in a similar way to pharmaceutical drugs known as calcium-channel blockers, but its diuretic action does not alter the ratio of sodium to potassium in the blood. Celery Seeds can have a calming and sedative affect due to limonene which acts as a mild tranquiliser and may help in treating anxiety, nervousness, mental stress and insomnia. Use caution in acute kidney conditions. Is a traditional Chinese medicine for hypertension, gout and diabetes. Useful in nervous restlessness and spasmodic tension, both topically and internally. **Contraindications –** Use with caution in acute kidney conditions due to the irritating effect of the volatile oils. Avoid in pregnancy and people with low blood pressure. **Part used -** Fruit (seeds) and root. **Constituents -** Volatile oil, limonene, Vitamins C, beta-carotene, sodium, magnesium and calcium, iron, potassium, zinc. **Dosage -** Tincture 2 to 4 mls 3 times daily. Infusion – 1 to 2 teaspoonful's of crushed seeds to cup of boiling water. Cover cup and infuse for 10 minutes 3 times daily.

Chamomile
Matricaria recutita

Actions - Antispasmodic, nervine, sedative, carminative, anti-inflammatory, analgesic, antiseptic, allergies.

An excellent gentle sedative with a relaxing action that is good for easing anxiety and helping with sleep. Helps to restore the nervous system. It is safe to use in children and is a powerful anti-inflammatory in almost any condition and a good all round tonic for the nervous system. This is the herb for those that can worry themselves sick. As a relaxant, chamomile depresses the central nervous system, reducing anxiety while not disrupting normal performance or function. Chamomile has been used for centuries to lower pain and reduce inflammation. This seems to be backed up by science with a 2009 study finding that Chamomile caused cell reactions similar to that of nonsteroidal anti-inflammatory drugs. In the digestive system it can be used for indigestion especially when there are colicky pains and is ideal for colitis and IBS type problems. For females Chamomile is good for amenorrhea, spasmodic dysmenorrhea, premenstrual irritability and menopausal tensions. This herb is also a good source of calcium and magnesium which are the nervous systems favorite minerals. **Uses** - Anxiety, colic, diverticula's, flatulence, gastritis, indigestion, insomnia, irritable, nervousness, cramps, restlessness, stress, ulcers. **Doses** - Tincture 2 to 4mls 3 times daily, for teas just the one teabag.

Comfrey
Symphytum officinalis

Actions - Demulcent, astringent, healing, expectorant, vulnerary, cell proliferant, bone healer.

Once widely cultivated as a fodder plant, sheep and cows eat it greedily so the plant was easily available to local populations who used it as a natural remedy especially in bone fractures. The impressive wound healing powers of comfrey are partially due to allantoin which stimulates cell proliferation and speeds the healing process inside and out. Also used in the treatment of diarrhoea, dysentery and shallow G.I. ulcers. These conditions respond to the demulcent, vulnerary, astringent and anti-inflammatory properties of the plant. The astringent action reduces haemorrhage associated with ulcers and colitis. Bronchial irritation and irritated coughs with hemoptysis (spitting blood) respond well. Comfrey tablets were even standard issue in World War II First Aid packs for the British as so widely known was the ability of this herb to speed up the healing of bones and wounds. It is very important to make sure that wounds are completely clean before applying Comfrey – this is because the skin can regrow so fast that it can trap any debris left in the wound, also bear in mind that the surface of the wound may heal and close faster than the deeper parts of the wound. Good for chronic varicose ulcers. Its old name is knit bone and that describes well what it does. Comfrey also guards against scar tissue from developing incorrectly. Used for all internal hemorrhages including uterine, reunion of wound and fractures, internal ulcers, ruptures, pulmonary problems, bronchitis, irritable cough, ulcerative colitis, skin ulcers and varicose veins. Comfrey is typically used to make compresses, poultices, ointments and salves to be applied topically. **Constituents** - Alkaloid (pyrrolizidine) (root only), mucilage, gum, tannin, silicic acid, phenolic acid (caffeic, rosmarinic, chlorogenic), allantoin, asparagine, choline, chlorophyll, Ca, K+, P, trace minerals, vitamins A and C. **Caution** - Short-term dosing only. 2 to 3 weeks on and 3 weeks off. **Precautions** - If taking Comfrey internally it is best done on the advice of an Herbal Practitioner due to the potential effects of pyrrolizidine alkaloids on the liver. Pregnant and nursing mothers should not use Comfrey. **Dose – Source from a Professional.** Tincture - 2 to 4mls 3 times daily. Decoction – 1 to 3 teaspoons full of dried herb into cup of boiling water for 10 to 15 minutes. Used as Ointment, Cream, Lotion, Fomentation, Compresses, Poultices, Washes, Baths.

Cramp Bark
Viburnum opulus

Actions - Nervine, sedative, astringent, antispasmodic, tonic, emmenagogue, dysmenorrhea, nervous system relaxant, anti-asthmatic, hypotensive, peripheral vasodilator, muscle relaxant.

As the name suggests this herb relaxes muscular tension and spasms. It has two main areas of use with the first being muscular cramps and the second in ovarian and uterine muscle problems. Cramp Bark relaxes the uterus and relieves spasms and cramps and was used in the past to help prevent miscarriages. The anti-spasmodic compounds in Cramp Bark work on all other types of cramps in the body including bronchial, gastrointestinal, genitourinary and skeletal muscle spasms. As a skeletal muscle relaxant, it is particularly effective for leg cramps. Its astringent action gives it a role in the treatment of excessive blood loss in periods and especially bleeding associated with the menopause. With spasms consider adding a supplement of magnesium as this could be deficient. Restores the sympathetic and parasympathetic nervous systems balance in voluntary and involuntary muscle spasms of the autonomic nervous system. Cramp Barks peripheral vasodilator action helps restore the blood flow to the arms and legs and helps to supply the magnesium that is needed. Cramp Bark is also rich in valerenic acid which is named from the sedative herb Valerian which was later used in the making of Valium. **Part Used** - Dried cortex (bark). **Combinations** - For the relief of cramp it may be combined with Prickly Ash and if severe Wild Yam. For severe leg cramps which won't go away add Ginkgo Biloba as it will open up the main arteries in the legs. For uterine and ovarian pains or threatened miscarriage it may be used with Black Haw and Valerian. **Precautions** - Do not use Cramp Bark if you have aspirin sensitivity. Not recommended for those on blood thinning medications. **Doses** - Tincture 4 to 8mls three times a day, for tea 2 teaspoonful's of the dried bark 3 times a day.

Damiana
Turnera diffusa

Actions - Nerve tonic, antidepressant, laxative, urinary antiseptic, stomachic.

Strengthening remedy for the nervous system, tonic action on hormone system, for anxiety and depression especially with a sexual association, tonic to the male reproductive system for impotence, anxiety and neurosis. Tonic for the aged especially in senile decay.

For males it is specially indicated for alleviating problems of achieving and maintaining erections. Damiana also works to relieve stress and anxiety related to fears of inadequate sexual performance. One of the active constituents of this herb is thymol which is a compound that is responsible for Damiana's life enhancing and stimulating effect on the mind and body. Used for mild to moderate depression, anxiety and nervous exhaustion. Its stimulating and restorative properties make it a valuable herb for anxiety and depression occurring together as can often happen as a result of long term stress. **Contraindications** – pregnancy. **Parts Used** – Leaves. **Dose** – Tincture 1 to 2 mls 3 times daily. Infusion 1 teaspoon full to cup of boiling water.

Echinacea
Echinacea angustifolia

Actions - Immune stimulant, anti-microbial, anti-inflammatory, alterative, healing.

This herb is an infection fighter active against strep bacteria (abscesses and boils), a blood cleanser, (blood poisons, snake bites, poisonous insects) and a glandular and lymphatic system cleanser. Use it particularly for respiratory infections and for any disease above the waist. This is one of our main immune boosters for the acute diseases. Echinacea stimulates the bone marrow to make more white blood cells which are our main infection killers and why we only use it in short bursts. Use as a prophylactic to protect from infections especially when traveling or before going into Hospital. **Uses** - All infections, depressed immune function, inflammatory conditions, allergies, effective against both bacteria and viruses. **Dose** – 1 to 4mls of tincture. **Warning** - Do not use continually as you will burn out the immune system, give a few weeks break after 3 weeks. Beware also in the use of allergies for you could be building up the immune system just to attack itself.

Devils Claw
Harpagophytum procumbens

Actions - Anti-inflammatory, anti-rheumatic, analgesic, sedative, diuretic, antioxidant, bitter and hepatic.

Specific for rheumatic and other joint diseases, arthritis, pain and muscle pain, lumbago, tendonitis, gout and inflammation of connective tissues. Devil's Claw is also beneficial in decreasing the progression of osteoarthritis by preventing cartilage degradation. Has a significant anti-inflammatory activity. Can also be used for tendonitis and to treat degenerative diseases of the musculoskeletal system. Affects the liver, stomach, joints, kidneys and is also a blood cleanser, removes deposits in joints, aids in the elimination of uric acid from the body. It is also a digestive tonic as the flavonoids and phytosterols found in Devil's Claw are antioxidant and stimulate bile production and is also an antispasmodic which may help in tummy cramps. The German Commission has given its approval on the Osteoarthritis and Digestive side. **Parts Used** – Secondary Tuber like roots. **Contraindications** - Caution with peptic ulcers and congestive heart failure. Not recommended during pregnancy or for diabetics, high doses can cause tummy upset. **Toxicity** - Higher doses may cause transient mild GIT disturbances such as diarrhoea and wind. **Interactions** - Less effective if taken with antibiotics (needs intestinal bacteria for activation). **Dosage** - As on bottle for capsules. 1 to 4mls of tincture 3 times daily.

Ginger

Actions - Carminative, diaphoretic, circulatory stimulant, sialagogue, vasodilator, ant emetic, anti-inflammatory, antispasmodic and mild anti biotic.

Ginger may be used as a stimulant of the peripheral circulation in cases of bad circulation, chilblains and cramp. In feverish conditions ginger acts as a diaphoretic promoting sweet and cooling the body. As a carminative it promotes gastric secretions and is used in dyspepsia, flatulence and colic. Reduces cramping, gas and nausea. Used for motion sickness. Ginger is good to mix with any other combination of herbs because it would help the body to assimilate those herbs and increase their actions.

Doses - Used in teas, tinctures, powders in capsules and my favorite crystallized Ginger which you can get in mild, medium or hot.

Hops
Humulus lupulus

Actions - Sedative, hypnotic, bitter, antiseptic, visceral antispasmodic, astringent, nervine.

Famed for its tonic and nervine properties, pain reliever, sleep inducer, antiseptic, tension that leads to restlessness, headache, indigestion, mucous colitis. Good for when digestive problems are caused by worry or nerves. One of the main remedies for IBS. Acts on the central nervous system and calms and eases anxiety. **Digestive System** – Nervous digestive conditions with insufficient secretions and over excitability of the nervous system. Visceral smooth muscle tensions affecting digestive and bowel functions, mucous colitis, spastic constipation, nervous dyspepsia, mucous colitis with Chamomile. Reduced stomach acidity and to check fermentation. **Nervous System** – Sedative to encourage restful sleep, insomnia due to worry or nervous debility with Valerian, reduces symptoms of nervous tension, nerve pains, excitability and hysteria with Valerian. **Doses** - Tincture 1 to 4mls 3 times daily, 1 teaspoon of dried flowers in tea 3 times a day or just before bed. **Caution** - Do not use in depression.

Licorice
Glycyrrhiza glabra

Actions - Anti bacterial, anti-viral, expectorant, demulcent, anti-inflammatory, adrenal tonic, anti-spasmodic, mild laxative, nutritive. Licorice improves macrophage activity and increases the production of interferon which is antiviral. Licorice extract also has broad spectrum anti-microbial effects along with being an antioxidant protecting the tissues especially those of the liver from free radical damage. The root part is used, licorice is one of our best demulcents especially for sore throats and painful and inflamed airways where it hurts to cough and is also good for gastric ulcers as it coats and soothes them giving protection and reducing the inflammation, it is also nutritive and slightly laxative. It contains the building blocks of hormones, has a marked effect on the endocrine system and the glands of the body along with catarrh, bronchitis, coughs, gastric and peptic ulcers and abdominal colic. Can be used for treating inflammatory and allergic conditions. A recent study at the Institute of Medical Microbiology and Virology, Kiel, Germany, researchers found that licorice extract produced a potent effect against strains of H. pylori which are the main culprits for Peptic Ulcers. **Uses** - Treatment of cough, inflamed throat, pneumonia, pleurisy, TB, all catarrhal conditions, gallstones, chronic constipation, arthritis, fatigue, female infertility, pains of colic, stress, easing gastric ulcers, inhibits the herpes simplex virus. **Interactions** - With diuretics, cardiac glycosides, corticosteroids, blood pressure medications, laxatives. **Caution** - Do not use with high blood pressure. Long term use can also raise the blood pressure. Better for use in formulas, minimal adverse effects if intake is less than 10mg/day. **Dose -** 1 to 3mls of the tincture 3 times a day.

Meadowsweet
Filipendula ulmaria

Actions - Antiseptic, analgesic, anti-inflammatory, astringent, diaphoretic, anti-coagulant, acid balancer, carminative, anti-emetic, digestive, hepatic, anti-rheumatic.

One of the best digestive herbs and is also known as the acid balancer. Containing salicylic acid Meadowsweet is an effective herb against inflammation along with having with other compounds in it making it much easier on the lining of the stomach. Has specific use for peptic ulcers both as preventative and for treatment, especially the chronic ones. Meadowsweet has been shown to inhibit the growth of the Helicobacter pylori bacteria. Used for heartburn, hyperacidity, gastritis and reduces fever. Regulates gastric acid levels and protects and soothes the gastro intestinal tract and mucous membranes. Its gentle astringency is useful in treating diarrhoea, especially in children. Of great use in musculoskeletal conditions such as arthritis, gout and all kinds of muscle and joint pains. It promotes uric acid excretion. **Parts used** – Aerial. **Constituents -** Volatile oil, salicin, salicylic acid (analgesic and anti-inflammatory), flavonoids, tannins, coumarins, mucilage. **Contraindications** – Avoid if you are allergic to salicylates or aspirin. **Dosage -** Tea 1 to 2 tea spoonsful in cup of tea infuse for 10 minutes. Tincture 1 to 4 mls 3 times per day.

Nettles
Urtica dioica

Actions - Astringent, diuretic, tonic, galactagogue, tonic, nutritive, anti-allergenic, anti-inflammatory, anti-septic, anti-hemorrhagic, hemostatic, hypotensive, nutritive, anti-rheumatic.

Is specific for nervous eczema and will strengthen and support the whole body. Plays an important role in chronic and degenerative conditions of the musculoskeletal system such as Rheumatism and Osteoarthritis, Gout, along with joint and muscle pain. A new study found Nettle Leaf extract had a positive effect against the genes associated with rheumatoid arthritis. Increases urine output and the removal of uric acid. The diuretic action makes it useful in the treatment of fluid retention, arthritis with swollen joints, and congestive heart disease. Specific for nervous eczema and children with eczema. Preventative against many ailments, hay fever, allergies, eczema and hemorrhage. Used in the treatment of wasting diseases, poor appetite, lung disorders, blood impurities and allergies. **Prostrate Problems** - Recent studies have found that Nettle is effective in reducing prostate size. It not only reduces the prostate size, it also alleviates the symptoms such as the frequent urge to urinate, painful urination and incomplete emptying of the bladder. Nettle leaf works well for inflammation of the prostate and other inflammations whilst the Nettle root is much better for BPH. Benign prostatic hyperplasia which means prostate gland enlargement. Nettles is an effective diuretic that can also help to break down stones in the kidney preventing painful conditions from worsening or requiring those stones to be either passed or surgically removed. **Precautions -** Hypersensitivity or allergy to Nettles may occur so start with a low dose. **Dose -** 2 to 4mls of tincture 3 times a day. Infusion 1 to 3 teaspoons full 3 times daily. Used as a tea from the leaf and or root. Taken in powdered root form for prostrate purposes.

Pansy
Viola Tricolor

Actions - Analgesic,diuretic, anti-inflammatory, anti-pyretic, anti-allergic, expectorant, alterative, laxative, diuretic, vulnerary, anti-rheumatic. Mostly used in three areas, the skin, lungs and urinary system. Specific for eczema and skin eruptions with exudates, especially with rheumatic symptoms. Can be used both internally and topically for any skin disorder with purulent discharge, psoriasis, acne and also for autoimmune diseases and edema. Topical use for cradle cap, diaper rash, weeping sores, itchy skin (Chickweed), varicose ulcers and ringworm. As a diuretic can be used for dysuria associated with cystitis as well as frequent and painful urination. Will also be of benefit in capillary fragility and easy bruising and atherosclerosis. For the respiratory system it will act as an anti-inflammatory expectorant for phlegm in the lungs, bronchitis and whooping cough. **Part Used** – Aerial. **Constituents** - Rutin, salicylates, zinc, saponins, mucilage, gum, resin. **Toxicity** - High doses may cause nausea and vomiting and allergic skin reactions. **Root** is emetic in high doses and has been used to induce vomiting in cases of poisoning. **Dose** - Tincture 2 to 4mls three times a day. Infuse 1 to 2 teaspoonful's of herb to boiling cup of water, infuse for 10 minutes. For our second herb we will use Meadowsweet again as it is a good back up for Pansy especially in the acid removal area and by this time you should of changed the diet so there should be less acid going into the system.

Schisandra

Actions – Adaptogen, immune stimulant, anti-inflammatory, liver and kidney tonic, restorative, nervous system tonic, mild anti-depressant, anti-anxiety and anti-stress, adrenal tonic, antioxidant, astringent, anti-tussive, lung tonic, regulates blood pressure, anti-cholesterol, sedative.

Of great use as a general liver protector that works well in the treatment of hepatitis. It is a liver detoxifier and works to deactivate free radicals that attack liver cells. Being extremely high in powerful antioxidants Schisandra helps to fight against free radical damage, thus lowering inflammatory responses. Can help in the nervous system by increasing the nervous reflex response and can also help in anxiety, depression, neurosis and stress. Promotes vitality and increases memory along with cognitive functions while providing resistance to stress. Is a powerful anti-anxiety herb lowering stress levels and enhancing mental performance. Because of its adaptogenic qualities it specifically reduces both mental and physical stress, exerting a normalising effect on the whole body. Schisandra reduces cortisol levels in the body (the stress hormone) and is effective in controlling changes in serotonin and adrenaline caused by stress. The herb is also considered a lung tonic because it helps the body to better utilize oxygen. Because Schisandra is high in powerful antioxidants it lowers the inflammatory responses, which in turn positively affects, tones and strengthens the immune system along with increasing physical performance and endurance and promotes recovery after surgery. Schisandra has long been used in the traditional medicines of China and Russia for a wide variety of ailments. As far back as 2697 BCE Schisandra was listed in the Yellow Emperor's Study of Inner Medicine, an encyclopaedia of healing plants. **Precautions -** Mild side effects may include indigestion, nausea, headaches and skin rash. Schisandra may promote contractions of the uterine muscles and thus should not be used by pregnant women. **Contraindications -** Avoid in fever. **Part Used -** Fruit (berries). **Dose –** Tincture 3 mls up to 3 times daily. Infusions - 1 to 2 tea spoons full to cup of boiling water 3 up to 3 times daily. Can also be found in powder and tablet form.

St John's Wort
Hypericum

Medicinal Actions - Anti-inflammatory, astringent, anti-viral, anti-spasmodic, nervine, vulnerary, antibacterial and antidepressant. St John's Wort is perhaps the most studied herb for depression with literally thousands of studies and clinical trials performed to assess its usefulness as an antidepressant. Many studies have found the herb to be equally as effective as traditional antidepressants but with fewer side effects in mild to moderately depressed patients. This is not meant to be used in major suicidal depression. Taken internally it has a sedative and pain reducing effect, which gives it a place in the treatment of neuralgia, anxiety, tension and general depression. Hyperforin which is a component of Hypericum can inhibit synaptosomal reuptake of serotonin, norepinephrine, and dopamine. It may take 2 to 4 weeks to notice clinical results when taken for depression. Useful in mild to moderate depression, anxiety, neuralgia and myalgia's and generally for pains shooting down nerve pathways. This herb is antiviral both internally and topically. **Contraindications** - Speeds up the elimination of many drugs and can interfere with MAOIs, SSRIs, narcotics and reserpine. Do not use St. John's Wort during pregnancy or lactation. **Caution** - Photosensitivity can occur in susceptible individuals. Fair-skinned individuals should take precautions when exposed to the sun and the elderly should use protective eyewear when exposed also. **Part Used** – Aerial and flowering parts. **Dosage** – Tincture 2 to 4mls three times daily. Infusion – 1 to 2 teaspoonsful of herb infused into a cup of boiling water taken 3 times daily.

Turmeric
Curcuma longa

Actions - Anti-inflammatory, antioxidant, anti-cancer, anti-microbial, antibiotic, astringent, circulatory stimulant, anthelmintic.

This was kind of the forgotten herb that has now rocketed on to the market. I think most of the old Western Herbalists decided they would just use Ginger as Turmeric comes from the same family. We will start with Arthritis where it is very helpful with pain relief due to its powerful anti-inflammatory effects, so it will help with Rheumatism to. Used also in Tendonitis, Bursitis and generally for any pain accompanied by inflammation. Turmeric's antibacterial properties can help to heal wounds and skin abrasions and also help in the pain of these conditions. Used for liver and digestive complaints where it increases liver function and helps with jaundice, also promoting liver function and bile production along with protecting the liver from toxic agents. Turmeric is also a useful digestive aid to relieve flatulence and to protect the stomach mucosa against ulceration and moderates insulin response. Turmeric has been linked to improving brain function, especially in the areas of memory and attention span, curcumin is one of the main active chemicals that have been shown to boost levels of the brain hormone BDNF, which increases the growth of new neurons and fights various degenerative processes in the brain. Being a powerful antioxidant which neutralises damaging free radicals, it also increases the activity of the body's own antioxidant enzymes and stimulates the body's own antioxidant mechanisms against free radicals which is good for heart health. Curcumin improves the function of endothelium which is the lining of the blood vessels. Endothelium dysfunction is a well-known cause for heart disease as it is what the plaques stick to and damage causing the blockages in the arteries. Curcumin interferes with intestinal cholesterol-uptake by increasing the conversion of cholesterol into bile acids by the liver which is another bonus to the heart. Turmeric can be an immune-booster and has also been shown to be cytotoxic to cancer and may be used to prevent and to treat cancer. This herb has been used in India for thousands of years, especially in foods and is one of the main ingredients in curry. As one of the main Ayurveda herbs it is used as a digestive, circulatory, and respiratory stimulant and is said to be cleansing for the chakras and purifying the body. **Constituents** - Turmeric contains Curcuminoids and a volatile oil containing turmerone, zingiberene, cineole and monoterpenes. **Vitamins** - Especially rich in B vitamins and C, B2, B3, B6 and Folate. **Minerals** - Potassium, Phosphorus, Magnesium, Calcium, Iron, Zinc, Copper and Manganese. **Precautions** - Turmeric can cause heartburn, stomach cramps or nausea. Take caution if you have gallstones. May also cause skin rashes in sensitive individuals and may increase sensitivity to sunlight in large doses. **Parts used-** Rhizome. **Dosage** – I have decided not to give any as all the dosages seem to be different and it is used in so many ways especially in foods, so follow what the label says as hopefully they will know the strength they are using it in.

Willow Bark
Alba

Actions - Analgesic, anti-inflammatory, febrifuge, bitter, astringent, antiseptic, anti-rheumatic.

Some people call this caveman's aspirin but the active chemical constituent salicin was only identified in 1829 by the French pharmacist H Leroux. This herb is used for a variety of conditions with the main symptoms being fever and pain. Salicin is a powerful anti-inflammatory and analgesic while other components of Willow bark have antioxidant, fever reducing, antiseptic and immune boosting properties. Used for mild flus and colds with fever, mild headaches and other pains caused by inflammation and used as a specific for Osteoarthritis and Rheumatism and other systemic connective tissue conditions with inflammatory changes such as anyklosing spondylitis, gout, muscular rheumatism, joint pain, osteoporosis, tendinitis, sprains, sciatica and neuralgia. This is also a good herb for heart health as it acts the same as aspirin but is longer lasting and it doesn't upset the stomach because it is absorbed into the blood via the large bowel so it prevents ulceration of the stomach and can be effective in reducing the risk of heart attacks and strokes. Antioxidant compounds called polyphenolic glycosides and flavonoids in white willow bark have been shown to protect against oxidative stress and various symptoms tied to aging, such as poor physical performance, cognitive decline. **Pharmacology -** Salicin is analgesic and anti-inflammatory. Is metabolized to saligenin in the bowels, then absorbed and metabolized to salicylic acid. **Toxicity –** Do not take if you are allergic to salicylates. High doses may cause gastric and renal irritation. **Interactions -** Avoid with alcohol, barbitutates or other sedatives, NSAIDs and anticoagulants. **Parts**

used - Bark (dried from 2-3 year old branches). **Constituents -** Mainly Salicylates with some others being beta-carotene rutin, tannins, calcium, iron, magnesium, manganese, phosphorus, potassium, selenium, zinc, B-vitamins, and Vitamin C. **Dose –** Tincture 5 to 8 mls 3 times daily. Infusion - Powder can be made into a tea, by infusing in boiling water for 10 minutes. Dosage 1 to 2 tea spoons of herbal powder to a cup of boiling water up to 3 times per day.

Withania
(Ashwagandha)

Actions - Adaptogen, analgesic, anti-tumor, hormone regulator, pregnancy tonic, rejuvinative, anti-inflammatory, sedative, anti-anemic.

Used to restore health to the nervous system and eases stress and mental exhaustion. Good for debility, nervous exhaustion especially due to stress and chronic diseases especially those marked by inflammation. Retards various aspects of the aging process and increases stamina. Promotes mental clarity and improves memory and stamina. Relieves pain by lowering serotonin levels which contribute to the sensitivity of pain receptors in the body. Tonic for the elderly and improves conditions associated with ageing. Promotes recovery after illness and during convalescence and has great use in various chronic diseases involving inflammation. Can aid bone degeneration, rheumatism, joint pain and neuralgias.

Dose - As on packet.

Introduction to Herbal Medicine

Herbal Medicine has been in use and developed continuously since the beginning of time. It mainly evolved from observations from what plants did and the affects they had on people along with their animals. There is also what they call the Doctrine of Signatures which works like this, that flower really looks like an eye, maybe it helps sore eyes? I'll give it a try as my eyes are so sore and red. You know my eye really feels a lot better now, I think I will call that plant Eye Bright (Euphrasia) and tell my friends all about it especially my Dad who gets sore eyes to. In this way hundreds of plants were identified that have a medical action and no doubt there were also a lot of casualties on the way. The next great leap in herbal medicine was the Roman Empire of 2000 years ago. The Great Armies of Rome all had their own Medical Corps with Doctors, Battle Surgeons and Orderlies. It was these men who already had the knowledge of the Greeks that started to put together the best medical manuals in the world while at the same time started developing and using medical instruments and tools, some of which are still used today. As the Romans conquered the known world more medicines and knowledge were found and assimilated. The next great leap was modern Chemistry which allowed us to see exactly what herbs were made up of and what parts of the herb causes its medical action. Drug companies have made billions of Dollars from this information as they find the main active ingredient and then make a synthetic version of it, one good example that we all know of is Valium which is the synthetic version of the active ingredient from the herb Valerian. Leaving aside the Drug Companies let's see how Chemistry changed the way that modern herbalists think. Modern science allows us to now know what Actions our herbs perform on the body so we shall carry on using Valerian as an example and see what Medical Actions of Valerian has on the body. The Actions of Valerian are Sedative, Hypnotic (sleep inducing), Anti Spasmodic (stops twitches, cramps etc), Hypotensive (lowers Blood Pressure) and Carminative (calms and relaxes the tummy especially if you are worried sick). Herbalists call Valerian the Herbal Tranquillizer and if you look at the actions you can see why, for if you can't sleep and your blood pressures up along with a gurgling tummy and an eye constantly twitching you definitely need to be calmed down. The modern herbalist is trained to think in actions. There are many reasons for this but the main ones are to stop them from just using a handful of their favorite herbs and to train the mind to work in the method of thinking in actions that are needed. If we start thinking in the actions that are needed for a patient it makes us consider the problem in far more depth than just using our favorite herb, and it forces our thinking to be far more holistic by taking in consideration the whole of the patient not just the part or the system we wish to treat. Let's take a look at thinking in actions. The patient has a cough, then the coughs can't stop and it sounds a bit like whooping cough. The patient also sounds a little hoarse and the temperature is also elevated. The actions that come into mind for this are expectorant for the cough, antispasmodics for the whooping quality of the cough and demulcents to sooth the sore throat. These are the obvious actions and we can add many more if we wish such as immune boosters for acute diseases, diaphoretics to reduce the temperature and prevent a fever and the list goes on but it's always best to keep it simple. Next we look at how Herbal Actions are used in making Herbal Formulas. Another point to make before we go to the formula making is that Professional Herbalists use Herbs in the form of Tinctures (water and alcohol solutions) as this allows them to mix formulas in any proportions that they like and also allows long term storage without spoiling. Along with using tinctures I also use herbs in powder form which can be a good and very cheap form to use and you can mix the powders into Herbal Formulas just as you do for tinctures but here you use capsules. If you want to use capsules you can buy capsule machines, some do 50 at a time while the ones I use do 100 at a time. I buy my empty capsules by the thousands but you could maybe start off buying 500 at a time with ebay being a good place to find them and the machines.

Making Herbal Formulas

You should never have more than 5 Herbs in an herbal formula otherwise you will start to lose track of what you are doing and how the formula is changing the symptoms. Always try to keep things simple. One of the herbs in the formula is used to force the formula into the body, to keep it simple we will only use three; they are Licorice, Ginger and Cayenne. As an example we will continue with the patient with a cough. After further study of the case we decide that this is an Acute Disease for it came on quickly and is fast acting and not slow like a Chronic Disease. Listening to the patients cough we decide that it is a dry cough and the patient has not got a runny nose. Let's list the actions to consider.

Expectorants - Licorice, Aniseed, Fennel, Garlic and Mullein

Antispasmodics - Aniseed and Fennel

Demulcents - Licorice and Coltsfoot

Immune Boosters - Echinacea

Anti-Bacterial and Virals – Garlic, Licorice and Echinacea

Out of the above I would choose Licorice, Echinacea, Garlic, Aniseed and Fennel. I would make the formula in this strength.

Formula

Licorice - 20%

Garlic - 15%

Echinacea - 15%

Aniseed - 30%

Fennel - 20%

These herbs are listed below. Read through them and consider why I used them, there are three obvious ones for Licorice alone with the first being to force the assimilation of the formula into the body. The second is for its expectorant action and third is its demulcent action in case the throat is sore and raw. Next time you see a little kid eating heaps of licorice, get them to open their mouth and look at their tongue which will be going black from the Licorice along with the throat etc, and know that you are looking at the demulcent action of Licorice working, by coating and soothing, and whatever it coats will also be getting its anti-inflammatory action as well. The most important reason that you use the Actions Method for Herbal Prescribing is so that you can concentrate the Actions which are most needed for example, if it's a Bacterial Infection concentrate on the Anti Bacterials, if it's a Viral infection concentrate on the Anti Virals and in this case when you look at the herbs below you will see that three of them have a expectorant action. Hopefully you are now beginning to see the importance of working in actions for if you don't concentrate a large part of the battle on the causes you may have lost the battle from the start. Read through all the Actions listed in Herbal Actions in the book and then do a study in depth of at least five Actions of your choice making the first two the Anti Bacterials and Anti Virals. Start trying to train your mind into thinking in Actions.

Licorice

Actions - Expectorant, demulcent, anti-inflammatory, adrenal agent, anti-spasmodic, mild laxative.

The root part is used, possessing unique pectoral and emollient properties; it is also nutritive and slightly laxative. It contains the building blocks of hormones, has a marked effect on the endocrine system, catarrh, gastric and peptic ulcers, abdominal colic. Its ability to soothe irritated mucous membranes and to break up phlegm and ease coughing sees licorice employed in respiratory conditions, coughing, bronchitis, and chest colds. Can be used for treating inflammatory and allergic conditions. Licorice has effects on the adrenal glands which are protective, restorative, tonic and stimulatory. **Uses** - Treatment of cough, inflamed throat, pneumonia, pleurisy, TB, all catarrhal conditions, gallstones, chronic constipation. **Dose** – 1 to 3mls of tincture 3 times daily. **Caution** - Do not use with high blood pressure. Long term use depletes potassium which raises the blood pressure. Don't use with steroids.

Garlic

Actions - Immune stimulant, anti-bacterial, anti-viral, anti-fungal, anti-septic, anti-oxidant, diaphoretic, cholagogue, hypotensive, anti-spasmodic, vermifuge and many more.

The plant is rich in volatile oil and sulphur and because of its remarkable penetrating, disinfecting and mucous expelling powers garlic is a valuable basic remedy for the treatment of all ailments in which the cleansing of the blood stream and expulsion of mucous accumulations is required. Garlic is one of our main herbs used to prevent and treat respiratory infections. Anyone who has had garlic breath has experienced this herb's aromatic compounds being excreted through their lungs, which is why garlic's active ingredients can be so effective for respiratory complaints. Garlic is extremely effective in dissolving and cleansing cholesterol from the blood stream, it stimulates the digestive tract, kills worms, parasites and harmful bacteria, normalizes blood pressure, reduces fever, gas and cramps. I use Garlic in oil form (Garlic Oil Capsules) for respiratory infections as the oil goes into the blood stream fast and a lot of it exits via the lungs hence the garlic breath. **Uses-** All infections, coughs, colds, flu, bronchitis, all fevers, pulmonary conditions, gastric and skin complaints, rheumatism, all worms and ringworm, ticks and lice. Acts on Bacteria, Viruses and Internal Parasites. **Dose** – 3000mg Garlic Oil tabs are the best way to go as it gets into the blood fast. For those who cannot tolerate the breath use Kyloc the Japanese aged form as this is odorless.

Echinacea

Actions - Immune stimulant, anti-microbial, anti-inflammatory, alterative, healing.

This herb is an infection fighter active against strep bacteria (abscesses and boils), a blood cleanser, (blood poisons, snake bites, poisonous insects) and a glandular and lymphatic system cleanser. Use it particularly for respiratory infections and for any disease above the waist. This is one of our main immune boosters for the acute diseases. Echinacea stimulates the bone marrow to make more white blood cells which are our main infection killers, and why we only use it in short bursts. Use as a prophylactic to protect from infections especially when traveling or before going into Hospital. **Uses** - All infections, depressed immune function, inflammatory conditions, allergies, effective against both bacteria and viruses. **Dose** – 1 to 4mls of tincture. **Warning** - Do not use continually as you will burn out the immune system, give a few weeks break after 3 weeks. Beware also in the use of allergies for you could be building up the immune system just to attack itself.

Aniseed

Actions - Antispasmodic, carminative, expectorant, parasiticide, antimicrobial, galactagogue.

This is a herb with many uses, some of the main uses are intestinal colic and flatulence, a good digestive tonic and appetite stimulant, a good expectorant and along with its antispasmodic action it can be used for such conditions as bronchitis and whooping cough. Aniseed has mild estrogenic effects and can be used as a good herb for relieving some of the symptoms of menopause. This herb has a reputation of increasing milk production in nursing mothers, promoting menstruation and also facilitating childbirth. It is also said to increase libido in men and women. **Doses -** Mainly used as a tea, 1 to 2 teaspoonful's of seeds add boiling water, cover and leave for 5 to 10 minutes.

Fennel

Actions - Carminative, aromatic, anti-spasmodic, stimulant, galactagogue, expectorant.

The herb possesses highly antiseptic and tonic properties. The primary use of fennel is to relieve bloating, but it also settles stomach pain, stimulates the appetite and is diuretic and anti-inflammatory.

Uses - Gastric ailments, relieves flatulence and colic, stimulates appetite, inflammation of the bowels, acute constipation (raw roots daily), fevers, cramps, worms, indigestion, all eye ailments, bronchitis, coughs, muscular and rheumatic pains use the oil. Externally used as an eye wash to treat eye infections. **Dose** - 2 to 4mls of tincture 3 times daily.

The more you look at the formula and compare it to the herbs I chose the more you will learn and see the different reasoning that was considered but do this over time when you have learnt more about herbs and are getting used to using them.

How to Make Herbal Tinctures

Tinctures are made by steeping the Herb plant material in a mixture of alcohol and water. Alcohol is usually always used at strength of 45%. The alcohol in this mixture will extract all the essential oils from the herb while the water will extract all that is water soluble, so between the both we are getting most of the medicinal properties out of the herb. The proportions of herb to liquid are usually 1 part herb to 5 parts liquid. So find a suitable container (I use a big one liter preserving jar with a good sealing lid) and put into it 100grams of your chosen herb and to that add 500mls of our 45% solution of alcohol and water. Seal the lid and shake well for about a minute. Leave the jar on the window sill so the sun can shine on the jar for two weeks. The jar must be shaken for at least a minute every day. After 2 weeks open and filter the contents of the jar. I use a large pouring jug into which I place a funnel and then place a coffee filter in the funnel and pour the jar contents through the funnel being careful not to let too much herb spill into the filter and block it up. When you get to the bottom of the jar you can crush the herb in your fist so as to extract the last of the liquid. After this is completed you then get your chosen storage bottle, put a funnel into its neck followed by a coffee filter and then filter the jug into the bottle so it is double filtered. Next we label the bottle, put the date, name and proportions e.g. 1 to 5 also state the recommended dose. Store in a cool and dark place. Most Professional Homoeopaths and Herbalists have access to pure alcohol so for them it is fairly easy to make tinctures while for the lay person they will probably have a hard time. An alternative is to use Vodka as strong as you can find it or find a way to twist the authorities arm into giving alcohol at 45%. Don't even try to get pure alcohol as it is dangerous and can turn people blind and they won't give it to you. Or in the case of my brother get a still.

How to Make Infusions

Infusions are a bit like making a cup of tea except we don't use milk. Infusions are used for the soft parts of the herb such as the flowers, leaves and fine twigs. The proportions for infusions are 1 to 20 e.g. 1 part herb to 20 parts water. Infusions are used for the more water soluble herbs. Infusions can be made from a single herb or from a combination of herbs and may be drunk hot or cold. The water should be just off the boil before being poured on the herb and if you are making an infusion of a herb strong in essential oils such as Peppermint always cover the top of the cup to stop the essential oils from escaping in steam while the infusion is brewing. Allow up to 10 minutes to brew. It is best to make herbal teas fresh each day. You can experiment on yourself by getting Chamomile and Peppermint tea bags from the supermarket. Use honey as a sweetener.

How to Make Decoctions

Decoctions are used for the more hard woody substances of the herb such as barks, berries or roots. The process of decoction is far more vigorous then infusion as it involves heating the plant material in cold water, bringing it to the boil and simmering for 20 to 40 minutes. The finished ratio for decoctions is again 1 part herb to 20 parts water; remember to add more water at the beginning so you wind up with the 1 to 20 after steam loss. This form of preparation is no good for the herbs that are high in essential oils as these will all be lost in the steam.

How to Make Your Own Creams

Herbal Tinctures for medicating creams will be Calendula, St John's Wort (Hyrpericum), Arnica and Witch Hazel. Use Comfrey and Castor Oil as and when needed. Find a good cheap seconds shop and look for Vitamin E or Lanolin cream in a really big jar so that you can fill lots of normal sized jars. For a normal sized jar use half to three quarters of a small teaspoon full of tincture poured on top of a cream filled jar. We will do a hard one first which is the mixture of Calendula and Hypericum tinctures which are two of our best wound healers mixed together. Calendula heals and closes wounds fast (so make sure they are clean) while Hypericum is more the pain killer, antiseptic and tetanus prevention. To make this easier find a small 10 to 15ml bottle and label it Hypercal and fill it half and half of each so from now on you have a bottle of Hyercal. Next fill a normal sized jar fill of your chosen cream then bang the base of the jar fairly hard twice on the kitchen table which should settle all the cream to the bottom of the jar, if it looks as though it needs more cream repeat the process. Get a small teaspoon and three quarter fill it and pour on the cream. Next turn the teaspoon upside down and use the handle to stir the cream in the jar. After two and a half minutes of stirring you will start thinking this isn't working. After five minutes you will think there it goes. Some creams are faster than others but most take a lot of stirring. This is the way we medicate creams. When doing this get to know the herb, smell it, then put a drop on your finger and taste it. Is it really bitter? If so it will be a good digestive herb, get to know your new friends. As we age and get older the skin becomes thinner so we become prone to more injuries especially on the hands. Every year I would always give my parents a big jar of Hypercal for Christmas and at the end of the year it was usually close to the empty.

Cuts and Wounds

The first consideration is to stop the bleeding, rule out any deeper internal damage and clean and disinfect the wound. To stop the bleeding apply pressure. Calendula is one of the main lotions used for cleaning wounds as it is gentle, soothing, astringent, healing and anti-microbial so it kills the germs as well. Calendula has a tendency of sometimes welding the skin together (handy for closing knife cuts) this is more noticeable on wounds with clean cut edges. Because of this tendency it is very important to make sure that all wounds are very clean and no dirt remains inside. Now we will introduce you to Hypericum (St John's Wort), I use Hypericum lotion on wounds that are in very nerve rich areas, a good example is crush injuries to the finger as we all know how painful and sensitive a wound is to this area. As well as being used for nerve damage Hypericm is also astringent so it will help in stopping the bleeding and its anti-inflammatory action should help to reduce the swelling. I usually get a separate bottle and fill it up with half Hypericum and half Calendula tincture and call this bottle Hypercal. I use this bottle for making my lotions for deep wounds and on nervy areas. Consider also that these are both astringents so our power to stop bleeding has been increased. Tea Tree Oil is good for small wounds and has a strong antibacterial action but can sometimes hurt in open wounds. The oil is good where there is infection as it draws pus to a head. If you have a clean cut wound fairly deep but on the border line of getting stitches and have managed to stop the bleeding here's a way of putting a kind of skin graft on it which will hold the wound shut while you decide what to do but clean the wound first calendula lotion as this will sometimes seal it. Break and empty an egg. On the inside of the egg shell you will see a plastic like skin, peel this off and lay across the wound wet side down. The skin is also meant to have an antibiotic action which protects the egg. If you are going to try to get away without stitches try to immobilize the area for a couple of days so you don't accidentally rip the wound open again and use plenty of Calendula to close the wound.

Herbal Treatment

1. Deal with bleeding and clean wound under running tap water if possible.

2. Do the final cleaning with Calendula or Hypercal lotion mixed 1 to 20 parts water.

3. Cover and protect the wound if you think it is necessary.

4. When wound is dry and healing (if weeping use Hypercal lotion) you can use Calendula cream with maybe Comfrey cream as well for scar prevention or if the wound is healing slowly. You can also medicate a little bit of Calendula cream with Hypericum to make a Hypercal cream for a healing wound giving off nervy pain. Hypericum is the next most well used lotion, its main calling is for wounds of the very nervy parts of the body such as the fingers, tail bone, lips or for any part that really hurts and is nervy. One of the leading symptoms for Hypericum is shooting pains along the nerve pathways from the injured area. Hypericum is good for infections and septic conditions in nervy areas and I would use it with Calendula for any infection in a wound especially deep wounds. In the past Hypericum was used to prevent Tetanus in deep puncture wounds especially from rusty metal objects. Remember infections are trying to get the rubbish out of the body so when they begin to discharge do not try to stop the discharge let the body get rid of its rubbish.

Hypercal - Which is a half and half mixture of Hypericum and Calendula tinctures, you can use this to make lotions when you want the effects of both Calendula and Hypericum together. An example would be an infected crushed finger.

Creams- Calendula and Hypericum creams can be used when the healing begins and are applied for the same reasons as the lotions but always remember the lotion gets in better. Creams are more for the latter stages of healing.

Our Two Main Wound Herbs
Calendula

Actions - Anti-inflammatory, astringent, vulnerary, anti-fungal, germicide, demulcent. **Part Used** - The Flowers. **Used For** - Minor skin problems, cuts, abrasions, rashes, spots, acne, slow healing wounds, skin ulcers and to improve post-operative healing, fungal skin infections such as thrush, athletes foot and ring worm. Used to stop bleeding, heal bruises and sprains, skin ulcers, minor burns and scolds, healing, soothing, and anti-microbial. As a douche or bath to treat vaginal thrush. Gargle for sore throat and tonsillitis. It can be applied as a lotion, ointment, wash, gargle, compress, poultice, bath and douche as required. Use as a lotion (1 to 20) to clean wounds, one of our main germicides for wounds and if Hypericum is added to the lotion you may prevent tetanus as well. **Caution** - Calendula closes wounds rapidly so make sure they are very clean and no foreign bodies remain. **How To Use** – For a very serious wound bleeding medicate a cloth with tincture and apply with pressure to the area till bleeding stops. Use as a Lotion one part tincture to twenty parts water to wash out wounds or medicate affected area, make at 1 to 10 for bleeding or fungal infections. Use a teaspoon of tincture to medicate a small jar of cream then stir rapidly for 5 minutes or less if it mixes in fast, usually they don't. I usually get a cheap Vitamin E cream from one of the big cheap wholesalers and medicate the cream with Calendula. Use Tincture for medicating creams. **Herbal Actions of Calendula - Germicide** - Calendula is a strong antiseptic, due to it wide variety of chemical constituents, including carotenoids which speed up wound healing and strengthens cells. Along with fighting bacteria in topical preparations, Calendula also fights viruses and fungi, particularly those on the skin and nails. **Anti-inflammatory**- Where-ever there is skin irritation and redness an anti-inflammatory action is needed to help the skin recover. With Calendula also being a Germicide it takes out the cause of the inflammation which is usually infection. Here the triterpenealcohols in Calendula exert their powerful inflammation reducing effects. They contribute to the plants overall ability to heal wounds such as burns, cuts and grazes as effectively or more effectively than conventional steroidal applications. **Astringent** - The most important use of the astringents in First Aid is to stop the bleeding and they do this by causing the arterioles and arteries to spasm at the cut end. Calendula is well known for stopping bleeding especially in the hard to stop areas such as the palms of hands where in the serious cases tinctures can be used on cloth and put in the palm and the patient made to make a fist. Calendulas astringent action can be used to improve blood vessels and tone and tighten up skin cells, thus reducing the occurrence of complaints such as hemorrhoids. (Use with Witchazel and Hypericum). Many new mums find themselves looking for a natural way to combat this condition and it is important to do so as there is a risk of developing blood clots. **Demulcent**- The soothing properties of Calendula are due to many of its chemical constituents in particular the triterpene saponins and mucilage. Both of these substances provide a soft and soothing healing effect on external skin surfaces.

Hypericum - (St John's Wort)

Medicinal Actions- Anti-inflammatory, astringent, anti-viral, anti-spasmodic, nervine, vulnerary, antibacterial. **Part Used** - Aerial parts. **Uses** –For First Aid we are concentrating on external use only. Used for wounds with pains that shoot along the nerves in nerve rich areas such as the fingers, lips, tail bone and toes. As a lotion it will speed the healing of wounds and bruises and is used where there is nerve damage and the possibility of tetanus. The main remedy for puncture wounds as it can sometimes kill tetanus. Good for varicose veins especially the painful kind and mild burns. Patients recovering from surgery where the nerves have been damaged often recover faster with Hypericum. For inflamed joints and rheumatic pain, painful abscesses, bad insect stings, damaged nerves from impact injuries, sprains and ulcers. Eases the pain in conditions such as lumbago, sciatica and Shingles (antiviral) where a cream can be used on the sore and the oil applied along the affected nerve path. As a lotion it is commonly mixed with Calendula, Homoeopaths call this lotion Hypercal. **How To Use -** Use as a Lotion one part tincture to twenty parts water to wash out wounds or medicate affected area, make at 1 to 10 for painful and dirty wounds. Mix with Calendula in large painful bleeding wounds with a chance of tetanus. Use Tincture for medicating creams. In **1907 Ellingwood** a famous Herbalist of the time listed the uses for muscular bruises, deep soreness, painful parts, and a sensation of throbbing in the body without fever. Burning pain or deep soreness of the spine upon pressure, spinal irritation and circumscribed areas of intense soreness over the spinal cord or ganglia. Concussion shock or injury to the spine, lacerated or punctured wounds in any location, accompanied with great pain. In the times of horse and carriages Homoeopaths were using it on horses to prevent tetanus after injuries to the hoofs mainly from puncture wounds from nails or similar objects as these wounds on the hoof were prone to tetanus. Hypericum has been one of the main Homoeopathic First Aid Remedies for hundreds of years used alone or mixed with Calendula in a solution called HYPERCAL. After the 1930's it faded from popularity but was used by the Russians in WW2 as a replacement for morphine in Lotion and Potencies. **Hypercal -** Hypercal is a 50 50 mixture of Hypericum and Calendula Tinctures. This is a combination of two of the best wound healing herbs mixed together. Calendula is more for dealing with the blood vessels and bleeding along with the rapid closure of the wound so care must be taken to ensure the wound is clean and no foreign bodies are there to be sealed in. Hypericums work is more on the damaged nerves and pain as well as infections in and of the nervous system especially those caused by deep and painful puncture wounds which could harbor tetanus if not properly cleaned and dealt with. By using these two herbs together you are doubling their main actions of anti-inflammatory and astringents with the last action being good for stopping bleeding and also infection. Wounds calling for Hypercal are usually bloody and painful. Works well on long and extensive grazes and cleaning gravel rash and wounds but is mainly called for impact injuries to the lips, fingers or toes. Ideal for closing clean incisions fast and after surgical operations. So the leading symptoms for Hypercal are painful wounds. Use as a lotion at one part to ten or 1 to 20 depending on your judgment of pain and infection. In emergency bleeding use the tincture as this will spasm the arterioles but be aware that the high alcohol content will cause pain in its raw state. Use Tincture for medicating creams.

Burns

The usual rule is to place the burnt area under cold water as soon as possible. I usually leave it under there till it's nearly numb from the cold. The point to remember here is that when you take let's say your hand away from whatever burnt it the heat from the burn is still traveling inward and will continue to do so for about 15 seconds so this is why you must get to the cold water fast so you can reduce the severity and the depth of the burn. For minor burns and scolds Aloe Vera gel straight from the plants leaf can give quick relief and speed up the healing. In Herbal Medicine we use astringents for burns (with the exception being for burns that cover a very large area) as the tannins in the herbs will seal and protect the burned surface. Tannins also have an antibacterial action so this should help in the prevention of infections. Deep burns always require prompt medical attention. **Herbal Treatment - Aloe Vera** - apply to burn straight from the plant. **Witch Hazel** - Use as a lotion at about 1 to 20 strength and apply to the burn, this herb is a strong astringent and should seal and protect the surface. **Hypericum** - This can be added to the above lotion as it has some similar actions but for burns we are mainly using it to reduce the pain. Once the healing has begun you can continue applying **Aloe Vera** especially if there is still pain. Another good herb for around the edges of the burn as it heals is **Calendula Cream**.

Understanding Homoeopathy

Homoeopathy has been around now for hundreds of years and unlike most other forms of medicine its rules have not changed and will not for they are an essential truth. The main rule is Like cures Like or if we break down the word Homoeopathy homo means the same and pathy means disease. As Homoeopathy is a very hard science to learn and as it kind of sits or balances on the boarder of hard science and metaphysics I will not try to explain to you in detail what it is here, as it would probably take a whole book to do this but I will say this, in the UK and a lot of countries in Europe and especially in India it is on and paid for by the National Health Systems and anything that can get a politician to open their purse must have a lot of truth in it. It is said that Homoeopathy sits on a three legged stool. What this means is that if a remedy has at least three symptoms in the same strength as your patients symptoms, then that remedy is a potential cure for their condition or if not cure it will offer relief. The more symptoms you can match to the remedy the better the remedy will work for the rule is likes cure likes not vaguely similar cures. Listed below is an example of a Homoeopathic remedy from William Boerickes Materia Medica and some of the symptoms it covers. The idea is to find one remedy that covers most of your symptoms. Pay special notice of the Mental symptoms as these are some of the most important symptoms to try to match. Notice the way it set out, the italic writing says that these symptoms are strong in the remedy. This is a very common remedy in Homoeopathy and is known as one of the Polycrests, you will see it in many of the diseases so come back here to refer to it. Relating to Dementia we can see two good symptoms in the **Mind** area with the first being Hallucinations and the next, Sensitive to disorder and confusion. Look down towards the end at **Modalities**, these tell you what makes the condition better or worse.

Arsenicum Album

A profoundly acting remedy on every organ and tissue. Its clear-cut characteristic symptoms and correspondence too many severe types of disease make its homeopathic employment constant and certain. Its general symptoms often alone lead to its successful application. Among these the all-prevailing debility, exhaustion, and *restlessness*, with *nightly aggravation*, are most important. *Great exhaustion after the slightest exertion.* This, with the peculiar irritability of fiber, gives the characteristic *irritable weakness. Burning pains.* Unquenchable thirst. Burning relieved by heat. *Seaside complaints* (*Nat mur; Aqua Marina*). Injurious effects of fruits, especially more watery ones. Gives quiet and ease to the last moments of life when given in high potency. *Fear fright and worry.* Green discharges. Infantile Kala-azar (Dr. Neatby). *Ars* should be thought of in ailments from alcoholism, *ptomaine poisoning*, stings, dissecting wounds, chewing tobacco; ill effects from decayed food or animal matter; odor of discharges is *putrid*; in complaints that return annually. Anemia and chlorosis. Degenerative changes. Gradual loss of weight from impaired nutrition. Reduces the refractive index of blood serum (also *China* and *Ferr phos*). Maintains the system under the stress of malignancy regardless of location. Malarial cachexia. *Septic infections and low vitality.*

Mind - *Great anguish and restlessness. Changes place continually. Fears,* of death, of being left alone. Great fear, with cold sweat. Thinks it useless to take medicine. Suicidal. Hallucinations of smell and sight. Despair drives him from place to place. Miserly, malicious, selfish, lacks courage. General sensibility increased (*Hep*). Sensitive to disorder and confusion.

Head - Headaches relieves by cold, other symptoms worse. Periodical burning pains, with *restlessness*; with cold skin. Hemicrania, with icy feeling of scalp and great weakness. Sensitive head in open air. Delirium tremens; cursing and raving; vicious. Head is in constant motion. Scalp *itches* intolerably; circular patches of bare spots; rough, dirty, sensitive, and covered with dry scales; nightly burning and itching; dandruff. Scalp very sensitive; cannot brush hair.

Eyes - *Burning in eyes, with acrid lachrymation.* Lids red, ulcerated, scabby, scaly, granulated. Edema *around* eyes. External inflammation, with extreme painfulness; *burning, hot,* and excoriating lachrymation. Corneal ulceration. *Intense photophobia*; better external warmth. Ciliary neuralgia, with fine burning pain.

Ears - Skin within, raw and burning. *Thin, excoriating, offensive* otorrhœa. Roaring in ears, during a paroxysm of pain.

Nose - *Thin, watery, excoriating* discharge. Nose feels *stopped up.* Sneezing *without* relief. Hay-fever and coryza; worse in open air; better indoors. *Burning* and bleeding. Acne of nose. Lupus.

Face - Swollen, pale, yellow, *cachectic,* sunken, cold, and covered with sweat (*Acetic acid*). Expression of agony. Tearing *needle-like* pains; burning. Lips black, livid. Angry, circumscribed flush of cheeks.

Mouth - Unhealthy, easily-bleeding gums. Ulceration of mouth with dryness and burning heat. Epithelioma of lips. Tongue dry, clean, and red; stitching and burning pain in tongue, ulcerated with blue color. Bloody saliva. Neuralgia of teeth; feel long and very sore; worse after midnight; better warmth. Metallic taste. *Gulping up of burning water.*

Throat - Swollen, edematous, constricted, *burning,* unable to swallow. Diphtheritic membrane, looks dry and wrinkled.

Stomach - *Cannot bear the sight or smell of food. Great thirst; drinks much, but little at a time.* Nausea, retching, vomiting, after eating or drinking. Anxiety in pit of stomach. *Burning pain.* Craves acids and coffee. Heartburn; gulping up of acid and bitter substances which seem to excoriate the throat. Long-lasting eructation's. Vomiting of blood, bile, green mucus, or brown-black mixed with blood. Stomach extremely irritable; seems raw, as if torn. Gastralgia from slightest food or drink. Dyspepsia from vinegar, acids, ice-cream, ice-water, tobacco. Terrible fear and dyspnœa, with gastralgia; also faintness, icy coldness, great exhaustion. Malignant symptoms. Everything swallowed seems to lodge in the œsophagus, which seems as if closed and nothing would pass. *Ill effects of vegetable diet, melons, and watery fruits generally.* Craves milk.

Abdomen - Gnawing, burning pains like coals of fire; relieved by heat. *Liver and spleen enlarged and painful.* Ascites and anasarca. Abdomen swollen and painful. Pain as from a wound in abdomen on coughing.

Rectum - Painful, spasmodic protrusion of rectum. Tenesmus. *Burning* pain and pressure in rectum and anus.

Stool - *Small, offensive, dark, with much prostration. Worse at night, and after eating and drinking;* from chilling stomach, alcoholic abuse, spoiled meat. Dysentery dark, bloody, very offensive. Cholera, with intense agony, prostration, and burning thirst. Body cold as ice (*Verat*). Hæmorrhoids burn like fire; relieved by heat. Skin excoriated about anus.

Urine - Scanty, burning, involuntary. Bladder as if paralysed. *Albuminous.* Epithelial cells; cylindrical clots of fibrin and globules of pus and blood. After urinating, feeling of weakness in abdomen. Bright's disease. Diabetes.

Female - Menses too profuse and too soon. Burning in ovarian region. Leucorrhœa, acrid, burning, offensive, thin. Pain as from red-hot wires; worse least exertion; causes great fatigue; better in warm room. *Menorrhagia.* Stitching pain in pelvis extending down the thigh.

Respiratory - Unable to lie down; fears suffocation. Air-passages constricted. Asthma worse midnight. Burning in chest. Suffocative catarrh. Cough worse after midnight; worse lying on back. Expectoration *scanty, frothy. Darting pain through upper third of right lung.* Wheezing respiration. Hæmoptysis with pain between shoulders; burning heat all over. Cough dry, as from sulphur fumes; *after drinking.*

Heart - Palpitation, pain, dyspnœa, faintness. Irritable heart in smokers and tobacco-chewers. *Pulse more rapid in morning (Sulph).* Dilatation. Cyanosis. Fatty degeneration. Angina pectoris, with pain in neck and occiput.

Back - Weakness in small of back. Drawing in of shoulders. Pain and burning in back (*Oxal ac*).

Extremities - Trembling, twitching, spasms, weakness, heaviness, uneasiness. Cramps in calves. Swelling of feet. Sciatica. Burning pains. Peripheral neuritis. Diabetic gangrene. Ulcers on heel (*Cepa; Lamium*). Paralysis of lower limbs with atrophy.

Skin - Itching, burning, swellings; œdema, eruption, papular, *dry, rough, scaly; worse cold* and scratching. Malignant pustules. Ulcers with offensive discharge. Anthrax. Poisoned wounds. Urticaria, with burning and restlessness. *Psoriasis.* Scirrhus. Icy coldness of body. Epithelioma of the skin. Gangrenous inflammations.

Sleep - Disturbed, anxious, restless. Must have head raised by pillows. Suffocative fits during sleep. Sleeps with hands over head. Dreams are full of care and fear. Drowsy, sleeping sickness.

Fever - High temperature. *Periodicity marked with adynamia.* Septic fevers. *Intermittent. Paroxysms incomplete, with marked exhaustion. Hay-fever.* Cold sweats. Typhoid, not too early; often after Rhus. Complete exhaustion. Delirium; worse after midnight. Great restlessness. Great heat about 3 am.

Modalities - *Worse*, wet weather, after midnight; from cold, cold drinks, or food. Seashore. Right side. *Better* from heat; from head elevated; warm drinks.

Complementary: *Rhus; Carbo; Phos. Thuja; Secale.* Antidotal to lead poison.

Antidotes: *Opium; Carbo; China; Hepar; Nux.* Chemical Antidotes: Charcoal; Hydrated Peroxide of Iron; Lime Water.

Compare: *Arsenic stibatum* 3x (Chest inflammations of children, restlessness with thirst and prostration, loose mucous cough, oppression, hurried respiration, crepitant rales). *Cenchris contortrix; Iod; Phosph; China; Verat alb; Carbo; Kali phos. Epilobium* (intractable diarrhœa of typhoid). *Hoang Nan. Atoxyl.* Sodium arseniate 3x, sleeping sickness; commencing optic atrophy. *Levico Water--* (containing Ars, Iron and Copper of South Tyrol). Chronic and dyscratic skin diseases, chorea minor and spasms in scrofulous and anæmic children. Favors assimilation and increases nutrition. Debility and skin diseases, especially after the use of higher potencies where progress seems suspended. Dose. Ten drops in wine glass of warm water 3 times a day after meals (Burnett). *Sarcolatic acid* (influenza with violent vomiting).

Dose - Third to thirtieth potency. The very highest potencies often yield brilliant results.

Low attenuations in gastric, intestinal, and kidney diseases; higher in neuralgias, nervous diseases, and skin. But if only surface conditions call for it, give the lowest potencies, 2x to 3x trit. Repeated doses advisable.

Boerickes Materia Medica is the best one for use by the lay person; once you have mastered it you can move on to the many others. To make the remedies as closer a match we can we ask lots of questions like the ones below and after we gather all the answers we have what is called a good Symptom Picture which we then try to match as accurately as we can to a Remedy. Homoeopathic Repertories are used for matching symptoms to remedies but in this book you get the specific for each disease so try to match them as best as you can.

Symptom Guide Questions

1. Is there a sudden onset, what time?

2. What time of the day does the patient feel either better or worse?

3. What is the effect of motion? Jarring, walking, running?

4. What is the effect of drinking fluids? Prefers warm or cold drinks?

5. Is the patient thirsty or not at all? Sips or gulps?

6. Is the onset from exertion, overeating, weather changes, emotions?

7. Mental and emotional state of patient? This is most important.

8. Better warm room, warm air?

9. Better cool room, cool open air?

10. Respirations - dry or wet?

11. Expectoration - watery or stringy mucous, easy or difficult.

12. Is there coughing

13. Position - better or worse from sitting, standing, lying, lying on which side?

One of the main rules of Homoeopathy is the closer the match of the remedy the higher the Potency you use. Potency is a measure of strength and most of the remedies we will use will be in the 30th Potency until we get some experience, an example of how you would write this is **Pulsatilla 30C.** (don't forget the C on the end).

Remember as mentioned before Homoeopathy sits on a three legged stool. What this means is that if a remedy has at least three symptoms in the same strength as your patients symptoms then that remedy is a potential cure for their condition or if not cure it will offer relief. Go to the library and take out a book that easily explains Homoeopathy especially in the making of the potencies.

Homeopathy Dosage Directions

Select the remedy that most closely matches the symptoms. In conditions where self-treatment is appropriate, unless otherwise directed by a physician, a lower potency (6X, 6C, 12X, 12C, 30X, or 30C) should be used. In addition, instructions for use are usually printed on the label.

Many homeopathic physicians suggest that remedies be used as follows: Take one dose and wait for a response. If improvement is seen, continue to wait and let the remedy work. If improvement lags significantly or has clearly stopped, another dose may be taken. The frequency of dosage varies with the condition and the individual. Sometimes a dose may be required several times an hour; other times a dose may be indicated several times a day; and in some situations, one dose per day (or less) can be sufficient. If no response is seen within a reasonable amount of time, select a different remedy.

What to Do If It Is All Too Hard

Most of the time in my books you normally have a list under the disease of all the Homoeopathic remedies commonly used for them with a little write up on how they are different. If you are having difficulties especially in a chronic disease condition and are house bound most of the time, what I want you to do is go to a Professional Homoeopath or even better get them to visit you at home so they can see the patient in their natural conditions. What I would like you to get from this is a remedy that covers all of your conditions. While he is there I would also like you to get separate remedies for the other medical conditions or aggravations which you could use as and when needed as each condition flares up. I want to empower you and put you in control of your circumstances and lessen the burden. A Homoeopath that sees you at home gets a far better idea of your problems and how they affect your life and makes it easier for them to match you to the right remedy and also makes it easier for them to prescribe for other acute conditions that come around from the chronic one. Be aware that They will ask similar questions as I have already mentioned so have a good read of the questions list so you will know what to expect and are able to give them an accurate answer. Homoeopaths want to know your mind, sleeping patterns, what makes you feel better and what makes your condition worse; they are like detectives trying to piece together a picture of you in the present moment of time which is what we call a person picture. So think of these questions you will be asked.